A MIGRAINE SUFFERER'S COOKBOOK

FEELING BETTER WITH ADDITIVE FREE FOODS

by
Diane Meredith Bentley

edited by
Lori Bentley Law

back cover and family picture by
Lori Bentley Law

food pictures and front cover by
Diane Meredith Bentley

published by
TRAFFORD PUBLISHING

in cooperation with
Bendith Books

Printed in Victoria, Canada

National Library of Canada Cataloguing in Publication Data

Bentley, Diane Meredith, 1945-
   The migraine sufferer's cookbook : feeling better with additive free
food / Diane Meredith Bentley.

ISBN 1-55395-290-1

   1. Migraine—Diet therapy—Recipes. I. Title.

RC392.B45 2002   641.5'631   C2002-905383-8

TRAFFORD

This book was published *on-demand* in cooperation with Trafford Publishing.
On-demand publishing is a unique process and service of making a book available for retail sale to the public taking advantage of on-demand manufacturing and Internet marketing. **On-demand publishing** includes promotions, retail sales, manufacturing, order fulfilment, accounting and collecting royalties on behalf of the author.

Suite 6E, 2333 Government St., Victoria, B.C. V8T 4P4, CANADA
Phone   250-383-6864   Toll-free 1-888-232-4444 (Canada & US)
Fax   250-383-6804   E-mail   sales@trafford.com
Web site www.trafford.com   TRAFFORD PUBLISHING IS A DIVISION OF TRAFFORD HOLDINGS LTD.
Trafford Catalogue #02-1004   www.trafford.com/robots/02-1004.html

10   9   8   7   6   5

Dedication

To my husband Roger who is my "official taste tester", for always believing in me, and his love

To my son Wayne for his wise advise, always there to help, and love

To my daughter Lori for her support, language and technical skills, advice and love

To my mother for her love and always supporting me in everything I do

To my three grandchildren, Casey, Megan and Kayla for giving me such joy

To all my friends and family for their valuable advice and encouragement to finish this book and their belief that it would be valuable for those who suffer from migraine

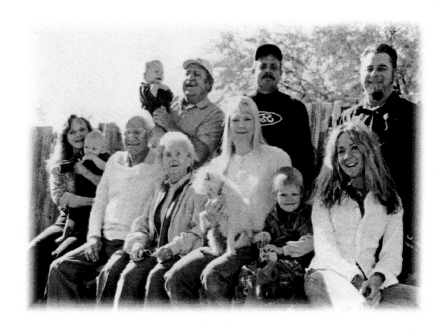

This book is also dedicated to my brother Jeff, who I loved to cook for, and I adored. My niece Kim, James and Jordan, my nephew Jeffrey, sister-in-law Frani and...Tony for loving us all.

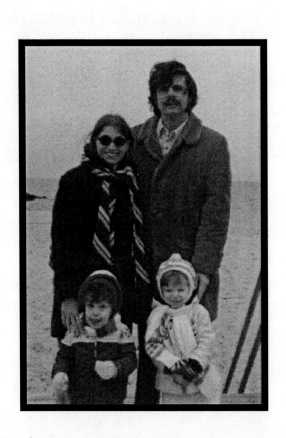

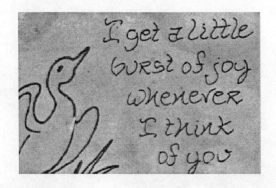

I get a little
burst of joy
whenever
I think
of you

TABLE OF CONTENTS

INTRODUCTION

I am a fifty seven year old woman who has suffered with migraine for most of my life, as did my grandmother, my mother and now my daughter. It's a genetic curse, but it can be helped.

I clearly remember my first migraine. I was visiting with friends, when a strange zig zag of light flashed across one eye, almost like lightening. Like a Salvatore Dali painting everything seemed surreal, almost as if the room were melting. People were talking to me, but I couldn't understand. Like an out of body experience, I felt disoriented and weak, my arm went numb and everything seemed as if I were looking through broken glass. Then came the pain. The awful throbbing pain that lasted for two days with no relief. I was sure it was brain tumor, so I went to a neurologist who, after much testing, told me I suffered from classic migraine. In 1970, migraines weren't taken seriously and there were no effective treatments. I continued to have them occasionally, maybe one or two per year, and that was tolerable, but as I got older the frequency increased to four per year, then once a month, and finally almost every day. It was becoming impossible to function and act "normal" at work. To try and explain to my co-workers that I couldn't see clearly or understand what they were saying would be impossible unless they had experienced migraine themselves. There were times when the symptoms were so intense, I couldn't remember even simple things, like my kids names. I couldn't speak coherently. I was afraid to drive anywhere for fear I wouldn't be able to get home. I had given up on doctors who prescribed drugs that were completely ineffective and had bad side effects. I resolved that this was my fate, that migraines were destined to control my life.

Then came the migraine that changed everything. A friend wanted to meet for lunch at a restaurant 35 miles from my home. Although I was nervous about the drive, I decided to go. En route, I began to get the flashes that precede my migraines. I pulled over to the side of the road to call my friend and tell her I'd be late. She understood my problem with migraine. Once my vision cleared I continued down the road but my tunnel vision left me so disoriented I barely made it there. I remember my friend waiting in front of the restaurant. I remember going in and sitting down but couldn't read the menu. From there everything gets cloudy. I remember being in her car, and sitting in a chair somewhere wishing I were home. I could hear people around me but couldn't understand what they were saying. Sirens were sounding and something covered my face. I was in an ambulance wearing an oxygen mask with an IV in my arm. My blood pressure was over 200 and I was admitted to the hospital emergency room where they gave me intravenous drugs. It terrified me. It terrified my family. After 10 more days of pain, I knew I never wanted to go through that again. It was time to find real help.

Through recommendations I found a neurologist who explained how migraine happens. She also helped me understand how critical food is to preventing future episodes, especially the importance of avoiding known triggers of which there are many. I followed the guidelines religiously, which not only included food issues, but also the importance of exercise, regular sleep, drinking lots of water, eating frequently and a drug regiment. It all made sense to me except the drugs. I've always believed in keeping my body drug free, and I was uncomfortable with the amount of pills prescribed. For me, the side affects of drugs aren't worth the benefits they may have, and while for some people they may be necessary I decided to base my treatment on food and exercise, not medication. However, you should always consult your doctor before making changes. Gradually I began to feel better, going an amazing two and a half months without a migraine. I thought I was cured and started eating foods that were "bad", and had three migraines in a two week period. That made a believer out of me, and I returned to the regiment of eating right and am feeling good to this day. The migraines are now infrequent and manageable.

The freedom from the pain of migraine changed my life. I wanted to learn as much as I could about food additives and triggers and so spent hours researching on the internet, reading labels in stores and experimenting with new recipes in my kitchen. I put together lists of natural products I had found, and discovered all the clever names that manufacturers use to disguise chemical additives. Before long, I had a large looseleaf notebook full of research and recipes and started thinking that others could benefit from the information I'd gathered. This cookbook was born from the desire to help others who suffer like I did and are ready to feel good again. I'm not a doctor, I can't guarantee it will work for you, but I can tell you that it changed my life! I can also tell you that food is a common trigger for migraine and through elimination of "bad" foods, you might be able to help yourself get better.

There are other triggers for migraine. I sometimes suffer when the weather changes. My daughter has hormonal migraines that come with her period. My mother would get weekend migraines, probably from the combination of stress from her job, sleeping late, and skipping breakfast. Migraine sufferers need regularity in behavior. One of the worst migraines I've had was on one of the happiest days of my life. After staying up all night witnessing the birth of my first grandchild, the adrenaline and lack of sleep caused a severe episode. Bright lights and strong smells can also be a problem for some. Ever been around someone with strong perfume and gotten a headache? Or had reactions to flourescent or flicking lights? Chemical household cleaners can also be triggers. I try to use natural products or make my own.. It's so easy and so much cheaper! You can find information on the internet or books on the subject. You can also find make-up, lotions, shampoo, etc. that are made with natural ingredients.

Migraine, to say the least, is a very complex disorder and there are no easy answers. Identifying and eliminating or lessening your exposure to triggers is the key to unlocking pain free days.

Through research, I've learned that twenty eight million people suffer with migraine, and that American industry loses around fifty billion dollars a year from absenteeism and medical expenses. Headaches account for about one hundred fifty seven million lost working days in a year. For those who suffer with migraine and chronic headaches, life can become unbearable. Some become so depressed and overwhelmed that they are forced to quit their jobs. But the good news is that there is help. You can begin by first visiting a physician for a proper diagnosis and by paying attention to your body and discovering YOUR triggers!

I wish for you many migraine free days!

For more information on migraine, visit the National Headache Foundation website.

WHAT ARE "BAD" FOODS?
AND
READING LABELS

Ingredients: Filling (high fructose corn syrup, fructose, glycerin, water, apples, modified tapioca starch, modified corn starch, cellulose, corn starch, malic acid, calcium phosphate, sodium alginate, cinnamon, citric acid, xanthan gum, caramel color), enriched wheat flour, sugar, partially hydrogenated soybean and/or cottonseed oil, whole grain oats, high fructose corn syrup, honey, calcium carbonate, dextrose, nonfat dry milk, wheat bran, salt, cellulose, potassium bicarbonate (leavening), soy lecithin, cinnamon, natural and artificial vanilla flavor, wheat gluten, corn starch, carrageenan, vitamin A palmitate, guar gum, niacinamide, zinc oxide, reduced iron, pyridoxine hydrochloride (vitamin B_6), thiamin hydrochloride (vitamin B_1), riboflavin (vitamin B_2) and folic acid.

THIS LABEL WAS ON CEREAL BARS FOR CHILDREN

WHAT ARE "BAD" FOODS?

Throughout this book I refer to "good" foods and "bad" foods. "Good" foods are additive free and should not cause problems. "Bad" foods contain the triggers that can cause migraine. It's amazing how many "bad" foods exist for those who suffer migraine. From canned soup, to low fat milk to bread to even the produce department, there are food time bombs. Keep in mind, not all of these foods may be triggers for you. Every person has a different chemical makeup and our reactions may be different. Chocolate is a trigger for me, however my daughter has no reaction at all. Peanuts are a trigger for my daughter, yet for me they are fine. To start, you need to eliminate all "bad" foods, and once you've gone migraine free for a period of time (2 weeks or more). Gradually add one food at a time to determine what your triggers are. The best way to determine what affects you, is to keep a food diary, like the one I've included in the next chapter. You must realize though, sometimes it takes several days to get a migraine from a particular food.

For some people, certain fruits and vegetables can be triggers. Listed below are some of the common triggers:

Fruit:		Vegetables:
avocados	kiwi	beets
bananas	mango	beans (all except for green)
citrus:orange, lemon, lime, nectarine	melons	mushrooms
dates	papaya	onion (use dried or powder)
figs	pineapple	olives
grapefruit	plums	pea pods
grapes	prunes	pickles
guava	raisins	sauerkraut
	rhubarb	

Avoid pre-packaged produce. Buying organic is always the best choice (chapter four explains organic). Or, better yet, grow your own.

Meat
Buy meat from your butcher since some packaged meats contain additives (or check labels very carefully).

Avoid meats and fish that are:
aged
cured
fermented
pickled
processed
smoked

Meats that contain nitrates:
corned beef
hot dogs
pepperoni
sausage
bacon
ham
processed lunch meats and canned meats (only buy tuna that says: tuna, water)

Bread:
You will be shocked when you read the label on most breads on the shelf. They are full of preservatives and unhealthy oils and even colorings. One of the best kitchen gadgets I ever bought was a bread maker. It's so easy and you have wonderful whole grain bread in a few hours. Most are programmable, so you can put the ingredients in the pan at night or in the morning and wake up or come home to the wonderful smell of bread baking. Some people have a problem with yeast. Don't eat fresh homemade bread right out of the oven, cool first and you shouldn't have a problem. The only all natural bread that I have found in stores is baguette bread. Not all of it is additive free, so be sure to read the label. Wheat bread, brown rice, whole wheat pastas are better for you than white.

Sweets:
maple syrup
molasses
licorice (candy, breath mints and gum often contain aspartame and/orMSG)
chocolate (contains a chemical called phenylethylamine that is a problem for many)

Cheese:
Many migraine sufferers seem to have sensitivity to an amino acid called tyramine found in stronger aged cheeses. I only use farmer cheese, fresh mozzarella, natural cheddar (white, no coloring added), Snofrisk cheese.

Nuts, seeds and oils:
peanuts, peanut butter, peanut oil
sunflower seeds, sunflower oil
sesame seeds and sesame oil
pumpkin seeds.

Coffee, tea, soft drinks, alcohol:
You should stay away from caffeine. If you must have coffee you need to know that some decaffeinated coffee uses a solvent in the process. You should use organic coffee that uses the "water method" of decaffeination. Caffeine is known to cause migraine (soft drinks, teas, coffee). Alcohol, especially red wine including wine vinegars can dilate the blood vessels in your brain and cause a migraine.

Sweeteners:
Aspartame (NutraSweet) causes MSG type reactions in MSG sensitive people. It is found in most products that say "sugarless" or "sugar free" such as diet drinks, chewing gum, breath mints, liquid medication, toothpaste, and even vitamins

Dairy:
I was eating low fat foods thinking they were healthier but low fat milk products (milk, buttermilk, sour cream, yogurt, cottage cheese, ice cream, cream cheese, margarine) often contain milk solids that contain MSG. It's better to use whole milk and real butter instead (of course, in moderation as they **are** high in fat) check the label on the butter though, as lots of brands contain coloring and added ingredients.

Speaking of **MSG (monosodium glutamate)**, let's get into additives and the importance of reading labels. First, a little information about MSG. Monosodium Glutamate is produced in the United States from sugar beet molasses in a fermentation process. It is a fine white crystal, easy to dissolve and very similar to salt or sugar in appearance, however, unlike salt or sugar it imparts no characteristic flavor of it's own.

4

The ever expanding use of MSG causes great concern in the medical profession because it stimulates brain cell activity. MSG "tricks" your brain into thinking the food you are eating tastes good. Manufacturers can use inferior ingredients and thus make the product seem tastier. Inferior products and higher profits prevail at the expense of consumer health. MSG is a poison to many people who are sensitive to its effects. During the past decade, a large amount of scientific research has been compiled on the effects of MSG in the body. Reactions range from mild to very severe. 30% of the population experience some symptoms from MSG in amounts commonly added to food. MSG intolerance is not an allergic reaction but a sensitivity to the chemical. Chemical sensitivities cannot be tested for in the same manner as allergic reactions, which is the reason for pointing out the difference between sensitivity and allergies. There are many reactions to MSG such as: headaches, migraines, heartburn, unusual thirst, stomach upset, nausea and vomiting, diarrhea, irritable bowel syndrome, asthma attacks, shortness of breath.

We have become a fast food society. Packaged "quick" meals are full of additives, a lot of which contain MSG. It is used in many restaurants and foods such as:

Bouillon, broth
Candy, drinks and chewing gum are potential sources of hidden MSG
Corn starch
Diet foods and drinks
Frozen foods
Potato chips
Protein and health bars and drinks
Salad dressings, mayonnaise
Sauces
Soups, canned and dry
Stock
Weight loss foods
Accent (is MSG)

For more information about MSG visit the NoMSG web site (The National Organization Mobilized to Stop Glutamate

READING LABELS

I was amazed when I started reading labels at how many products I would have never believed to be anything but natural weren't! Almost everything prepared is loaded with chemicals and ingredients you can't pronounce let alone define. A good rule of thumb is: if you don't recognize the ingredient, DON'T BUY IT! Don't be fooled by a product that says "all natural" on the label. READ the label, chances are it is NOT all natural. Re-check labels often as manufacturers sometimes change ingredients. **Below is a list of additives that may contain or do contain msg:**

Autolyzed yeast, yeast nutrient, yeast food, yeast extract
Autolyzed or hydrolyzed protein, soy, vegetable
BHA or BHT
Calcium caseinate, sodium caseinate
Carrageenan
Disodium guanylate and disodium inosinate (expensive food additives that work synergistically with inexpensive MSG).
Enzyme modified or anything "enzyme"
Flavoring, natural flavoring, beef flavoring, natural pork or chicken flavoring

5

Fermented, anything "fermented"
Gelatin (Jello) (capsules are usually made with gelatin)
Glutamate,monopotassium glutamate, lutamic acid,monosodium glutamate,MSG
Gums (guar, vegetable, xanthan)
hydrolyzed plant protein (HPP) hydrolyzed vegetable protein (HVP) any protein that is hydrolyzed, textured protein, protein fortified
Kombu extract
Malt extract, malt flavoring, barley malt
Maltoxdextran
Modified food starch
Nitrates or nitrites
Pectin
Pickled, preserved or marinated foods
Protease
Seasoning, seasonings
Soy and soy products (ie: soy sauce, soy lecthin, soy protein concentrate)
Spice or spices
Smoke flavoring
Pectin
Pickled, preserved or marinated foods
Ultra-pasteurized
Vegetable oil
Whey protein, concentrate, isolate

For more information go to www.truthinlabeling.org

These triggers are the common ones. Through research I have found that some people have problems with other foods like: wheat, corn, sugar, eggs, beef, and dairy. My daughter has a problem with cilantro. These are rare but that's why keeping a food diary is important. If you find you are still having problems after eliminating the common triggers, focus on other foods.

This list may seem daunting, but it becomes second nature to you as time goes on. For now carry a cheat sheet. If one of these foods is your favorite and you don't want to give it up, let me ask you this: Is eating a piece of chocolate cake worth a migraine? I think you'll make the same choice I did.

Now, what to do when you eat out? This can be quite challenging, but it is possible to enjoy a meal out. Avoid fast food. It tends to be high in MSG and chemical additives. Order simple foods in restaurants, like grilled meats or fish and ask to have it unseasoned. Add your own salt and pepper. Baked potato and steamed vegetables are usually safe. Ask for oil and vinegar instead of salad dressings that are loaded with chemicals. I actually carry my own homemade dressing in a small leak proof container in my purse. Take left-overs and healthy snacks to work.

This new way of cooking and shopping may seem overwhelming at first, but I've found that if you're organized and use the menu planners included in the next chapter to plan your meals for the week and the groceries you'll need, you'll not make unnecessary trips to the store. Stock your kitchen with the nonperishable items such as canned tomatoes, juices, herbs, spices, dried fruit, oatmeal, flour, sugar, rice, pasta and other items that you will use often. In Chapter Four I have included some additive free brand names and many phone numbers and e mail addresses to help you locate these products if you can't find them. Of course, by reading labels, you will find more products that are additive free. Be sure to add them to the list.

MENU PLANNERS AND DAILY FOOD LOGS

The following two forms are invaluable in my daily life. I suggest you make several copies and keep them handy.

Use the **MENU PLANNERS** to plan your weekly menus. For example, every Saturday decide what you and your family are going to eat for the week and the ingredients you will need to purchase. Planning meals will cut down on your shopping time and make your cooking much easier and organized. When shopping try to stick to the list.

There are lots of ways you can make meal planning and cooking easier. For example, when you make a sauce for a recipe, double it and freeze half for another meal. If you have a little extra time, do a little extra cooking for the week ahead. Prepare parts of the meal the night or morning before.

Be sure to eat three meals a day and three light snacks. Not eating regularly can trigger a migraine or headache. You should not go more than three hours without eating something. I have learned that protein and drinking lots of water is very important. Suggestions for snacks are: carrot and celery sticks or other vegetables, fruit, a small piece of cheese, lean meat or a hardboiled egg for protein. In the Snack section of this book try the Protein Drink, Healthy Snack Bars, Granola, Fruit Pops.

The **DAILY FOOD LOGS** are to keep track of everything you eat, which in time will reveal a pattern of what may trigger your migraines.

Be aware of the other "triggers" such as: weather, menstrual cycle, sleep changes, smoking, stress. bright lights, smells, missed meals. Make notes under the "other triggers" area if any of these occurred that day.

When you do get a migraine, you should circle everything going back 2 days. When you have another migraine, do the same. It will take several migraines to see a pattern.

USE THIS FORM TO PLAN YOUR MEALS FOR THE WEEK

S U N D A Y	BREAKFAST: LUNCH: DINNER: SNACKS:	GROCERIES:
M O N D A Y	BREAKFAST: LUNCH: DINNER: SNACKS:	GROCERIES:
T U E S	BREAKFAST: LUNCH: DINNER: SNACKS:	GROCERIES:
W E D	BREAKFAST: LUNCH: DINNER: SNACKS:	GROCERIES:
T H U R S	BREAKFAST: LUNCH: DINNER: SNACKS:	GROCERIES:
F R I	BREAKFAST: LUNCH: DINNER: SNACKS:	GROCERIES:
S A T	BREAKFAST: LUNCH: DINNER: SNACKS:	GROCERIES:

DAILY FOOD LOGS TO KEEP TRACK OF WHAT YOU ARE EATING FOR POSSIBLE FOOD TRIGGERS AND OTHER TRIGGERS

(weather, stress, menstrual cycle, sleep changes, smoking, stress, bright lights, smells, missed meals)

WEEK OF:_____

S U N D A Y	**BREAKFAST:** **LUNCH:** **DINNER:** **SNACKS:**	**DATE:** **MIGRAINE?** **OTHER TRIGGERS:**
M O N D A Y	**BREAKFAST:** **LUNCH:** **DINNER:** **SNACKS:**	**DATE:** **MIGRAINE?** **OTHER TRIGGERS:**
T U E S	**BREAKFAST:** **LUNCH:** **DINNER:** **SNACKS:**	**DATE:** **MIGRAINE?** **OTHER TRIGGERS:**
W E D	**BREAKFAST:** **LUNCH:** **DINNER:** **SNACKS:**	**DATE:** **MIGRAINE?** **OTHER TRIGGERS:**
T H U R S	**BREAKFAST:** **LUNCH:** **DINNER:** **SNACKS:**	**DATE:** **MIGRAINE?** **OTHER TRIGGERS:**
F R I	**BREAKFAST:** **LUNCH:** **DINNER:** **SNACKS:**	**DATE:** **MIGRAINE?** **OTHER TRIGGERS:**
S A T	**BREAKFAST:** **LUNCH:** **DINNER:** **SNACKS:**	**DATE:** **MIGRAINE?** **OTHER TRIGGERS:**

IS IT REALLY ORGANIC?

100% CERTIFIED ORGANICALLY GROWN

By serving Columbia Gorge canned cherries you can be assured that you have chosen the purest canned fruit available. From blossom to harvest and throughout the packing, this product is Certified Organically grown and processed in accordance with Oregon Tilth Standards and the California Organic Foods Act of 1990. This container is made of enamel plated steel and is lead free.

PLEASE RECYCLE.

For our earth & your health & pleasure,
Enjoy ...

INGREDIENTS: Pitted cherries, pear concentrate, water.
ALL INGREDIENTS CERTIFIED ORGANICALLY GROWN

IS IT REALLY ORGANIC?

I've never been totally confident that the products marked organic were really chemical and pesticide free.

Recently, after a decade of governmental wrangling and public debate, the USDA implemented national standards outlining exactly how foods labeled organic can be produced and handled.

Processors and growers will have a few months to become certified and implement the new organic production, handling, and labeling standards, and new labeling will take effect by October 2002. Independent certification agencies, designated by the USDA, will inspect farms, processors, and manufacturers to ensure that produce that wears the organic seal meets all federal requirements.

Once the new national organic standards are in place, consumers will begin to see three different labels, each of which is based on the percentage of organic ingredients in any given product. Only produce such as fruits, vegetables, and maple syrup that has been exclusively cultivated and processed according to the new organic standards will be permitted to bear the "100 Percent Organic" label. Packaged goods in which at least 95 percent of the ingredients by weight have been organically produced will be labeled "Organic". Packaged goods with 70 to 95 percent organic ingredients will be labeled "Made with Organic" and the specific organic ingredient will be listed. Products made of less than 70 percent organic ingredients are only permitted to list organic items in the ingredients panel and cannot tout the word "organic" in their primary labeling.

The three new organic labels guarantee that the products on which they appear do not contain any genetically modified ingredients and have not been grown using synthetic chemical fertilizers and pesticides or sewage sludge, a sterilized by product of municipal waste facilities that can contain traces of heavy metals like lead and mercury. Likewise, the products will not have undergone irradiation, a procedure in which food is bombarded with radiation to kill off bacteria and opathogen.

For more information visit www.usda.gov or www.ota.com, the Organic Trade Association's informative web site.

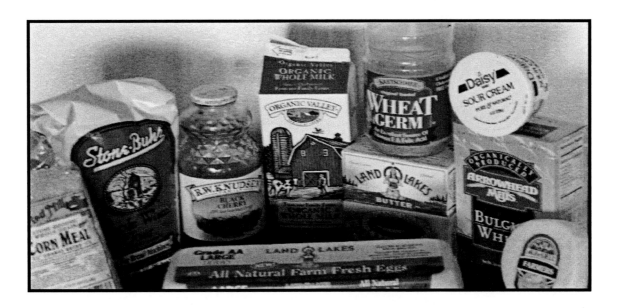

ADDITIVE FREE BRAND NAMES

The following pages list products that I have found to be additive free and easily found in my area. You may find them in some of your local markets or in speciality stores. Manufacturers change ingredients, so you should re-check labels from time to time. If you are not sure of an ingredient, check the list of additives in this book or call the manufacturer. A good rule of thumb is if you don't recognize the ingredient DON'T BUY IT! Some phone numbers and e-mail addresses are provided to help you locate the products in your area. A lot of these products can be ordered.

By reading labels, you will find other additives free brands. I've included pages for you to add the new products you find to the list and the store where you found them. Make a note in the product rating column so you know how well you liked them.

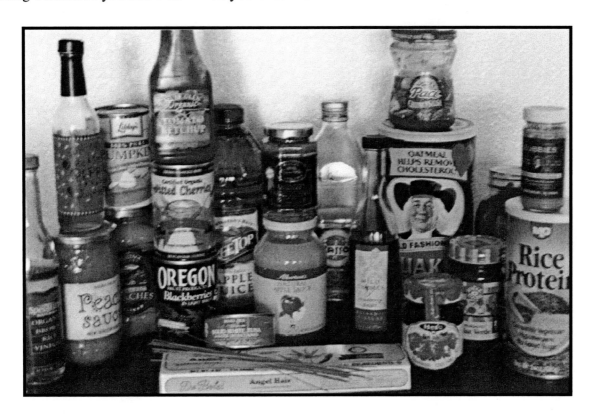

Beverages:	R.W. Knudsen - Just Cranberry, Black Cherry (knudsenjuices.com 1-530-899-5000) Martinelli's Sparkling Cider MLO Rice Protein (www.mloproducts.com) Mountain Sun Organic Juices-Pear, Peach, Apricot (mountainsun@acirca.com 1-866-492-5688) NutriBiotic Rice Protein
Bread For all your homemade baking: best to use Gold Medal All Purpose **Unbleached** Flour (or other unbleached flour) BEST TO USE WHOLE GRAIN FLOUR	A.J's Baguette French Bread Alvarado Street Bakery: Sprouted Spelt Bagels Arrowhead Mills Blue Corn Meal & Yellow Cornmeal CedarLane Fat Free Tortillas 100% Organic Whole Wheat (cedarlanefoods.com 1-213-745-4255) Fillo Factory, All Natural Fillo Dough Garden of Eaten Thin Thin Wraps Grissini Bread Sticks Starr Ridge Simple White Crackers/ Cracked Black Pepper (allen-cowley.com 800-279-1634) Tortillaland Uncooked Flour Tortillas (619-233-5139) Trader Joe's Baguette French Bread Whole Foods: Baguette French Bread, French Batard, Wheat English Muffin Whole Foods Organic Whole Wheat Tortillas and Red Chile Tortillas Willo Bread Company (602-254-0005
Cereals:	Barbara's Shredded Wheat, Puffins, Shredded Spoonfuls Kretschmer Wheat Germ Cream of Wheat Millstone Bakery Apple Blueberry Golden Oats Granola Nature's Path Oatey Bites and Honey'd Corn Flakes Pure & Simple - Puffed Corn and Puffed Rice Quaker Oatmeal
Cheese	Alp and Dell Farmers Cheese BelGioioso Fresh Mozzarella All Natural Cheese (belgioiosocheese@aol.com 1-920-863-2123) Cady Creek Farmer's Cheese Gina Marie Cream Cheese(Hilmar Cheese Company) hilmarcheese.com (or you can order it on: Cheese Express.com) all natural, contains no gums, stabilizers or preservatives (natural butter flavoring added at a very low rate and contains 99% water and 1% naturally cultured diacetyl. Manufactured the old fashioned way in cheese cloth bags, it is a three day process that includes turning and stacking the cheese cloth bags four times before it is ready for packaging. Friendship Farmer (some stores have their own packaged) Mozzarella fresh cheese packed in water may-bud Natural Semisoft Part Skim Farmer's Cheese (1-800-343-1976) Natural Cheddar Cheese (white) Polly-O Ricotta Cheese, Original (www.pollyo.com or 1-877-476-5596) Snofrisk Cheese (goats milk, cow's cream spreadable cheese)

Chips and Snacks	Act II Organic Popcorn Baked Pita Snax - Original Cape Cod Potato Chips Guiltless Gourmet Baked Yellow Corn Tortilla Chips Michael Season's Chips Olive Oil Potato Chips (goodhealth.com 1-631-261-5601) Organic Foods - Bearitos Tortilla Chips Padrinos Tortilla Strips, Restaurant Style Snyder's - Mini Pretzels Tassos Kalamata Greek Olives (1-800-4-TASSOS) Trader Joe's Mini Organic Pretzels, Shoe String Potatoes Veggie Stix (goodhealth.com 1-631-261-5608) Whole Foods Organic Peanut Butter and Almond Butter
Cookies & Desserts:	Breyer's All Natural Ice Cream - French Vanilla, Vanilla, Strawberry El Paso Chile Company Toasted Coconut (1-888-472-5727 Island Tapioca Kozy Shack - Rice Pudding Walker's - Shortbread Crisp Whole Foods Carob Powder (to make cake, icing and brownies) Wholesome Foods Organic Sugar
Crackers	Finn Crisp (www.vassan.com) Grissini Bread Sticks Ryvita Dark Rye Whole Grain Crackers Starr Ridge Cracked Black Pepper Crackers (www.allen-cowley) Whole Grain Naturals Yorkshire Crackers
Fruit	365 (Whole Foods Brand) Whole Cranberry Sauce Albertson's Natural Applesauce Adriatic Fig Spread, Lex Alexander (Whole Foods brand) Columbia Gorge Organic Fruit, pears, apricots, cherries Del Monte Peaches, Apricots (delmonte.com 1-415-247-3000) Eden Organic Apple Butter (www.eden-foods.com) Geisha Mandarin Orange Segments Heritage Fruit Hero Jellies:Blackberry, Apricot, Strawberry (123gourmet.com) Knudsen Organic Apple Butter(knudsenjuices.com530-899-000) Libby's 100% Pure Pumpkin (1-800-854-0374) Made in Nature Dried Apricots, Apples and Raisins Mariani Dried Cherries Mason Hill Farm Cranberry-Strawberry Jam Ocean Spray Whole Berry Cranberry Sauce Oregon Fruit Products (1-800-394-9333) S&W Premium Wild Maine Blueberries S&W Dark Sweet Pitted Cherries Saveur des forets Wild Cran Berries Solana Gold Seedless Blackberry Applesauce Sunsweet Cranberry Fruitlings Trader Joes Bing Cherries and Peach Sauce Trader Joes Sulfur Free Apricots Walnut Acres Jellied Cranberry Sauce (1-800-433-3998) Whole Foods Peach Applesauce Whole Foods Sulfur Free Apricots Wild Oats Sulfur Free Dried Apricots Wild Oats Sulfur Free Dried Blueberries 365 Whole Cranberry Sauce (Whole Foods brand)

Meat	Buy from the butcher and ask if they use additives or check labels on all pre-packaged meat Hans Mild Pork Italian Sausage and Golden Farms Sausage
Milk Products and Eggs	Alta Dena All Natural Heavy Whipping Cream (1-626-964-6401) Alta Dena Farmer's Style Cottage Cheese Small Curd Daisy Sour Cream (877-292-9830) Horizon Organic Half and Half and Horizon Organic Butter (www.horizonorganic.com or 1-888-494-3020) Land O' Lakes Half and Half (www.landolakes.com) Land of Lakes All Natural Eggs (www.landolakes.com) Lucerne Sweet Cream Butter Organic Valley Whipping Cream and Half and Half, and Butter (www.organicvalley.com) Trader Joe's Half and Half Vermont Butter & Cheese Company Creme Fraiche (sour cream) (1-800-884-6287) Vitamin D Whole Milk (organic, hormone free is best)
Pasta and Rice	Arrowhead Mills Couscous or Whole Foods Couscous Bifun Japanese Rice Pasta De Boles Pasta (1-800-749-0730) Eden Organic Pasta Company Parsley Garlic Ribbons (noodles) and Kamut Spirals (www.eden-foods.com) Lundberg Wild Blend and White Basmati (rice) Quinoa Pasta (elbows) Rivoire Carret Couscous Trader Joes California Rice Trilogy Trader Joes Organic Whole Wheat Penne Pasta
Sauces	Bubbies Horseradish Cucina Antica Roasted Pepper Sauce) Mrs. Gooch's Pasta Sauce (Whole Foods) Muir Glen Organic Tomato Ketchup (800-832-6345) Muir Glen Organic Black Bean & Corn Robbie's Sweet & Sour Sauce Parrot Brand - Roasted Garlic Salsa Sassafras Roasted Red Pepper Pizza Sauce, Spicy Southwestern and Basil Sun-Dried Tomato (Sassafras Enterprises, Inc., Chicago, Il 60612) Pace Chunky Salsa, All Natural Robert Rothschild Apricot Ginger Mustard and Raspberry Honey Mustard (1-800-356-8933) Whole foods Salsa Verde Whole Foods Salsa Caribe
Seasonings	First Choice Parsley Flakes and Chopped Onions Spice Hunter Spices (1-800-444-3061) Tones Ground Cayenne Pepper
Tuna and canned fish	365 Tuna (Whole Foods brand) Crown Prince Crab Meat Deep Sea Chunk Light Tongol Tuna Natural Sea Chunk Light Dolphin Safe Tuna Starkist Gourmet's Choice Tuna Filet Trader Joes Alaska Pink Salmon, Tongol Chunk Light Tuna Wild Oats Tuna

Vegetables (canned and frozen)	365 (Whole Foods brand) Super Sweet White Corn (frozen) (W Albuquerque Tortilla Company Frozen Red and Green Chiles (albuquerquetortilla.com) Castella Artichoke Hearts Contadina Tomato Paste Del Monte Whole Green Beans (delmonte.com 1-415-247-3000) Eden Organic Crushed and Diced Tomatoes (www.eden-foods.com) Green Giant French Style Green Beans, White Shoepeg Corn LaPas Sweet Roasted Peppers Melissa's Dried Tomatoes (1-800-588-0151) Muir Glen Organic Tomato Sauce (www.muirglen.com or 1-800-832-6345) Trader Joes Dried Roma Tomatoes Zorba Natural Pepperoncini (sulfite free)
Vinegar & Oil	Consorzio Oils: Roasted Pepper Olive Oil, Basil, Garlic, Rosemary (1-800-288-1089) Nakano Rice Vinegar Sasso Extra Virgin Olive Oil (this is a premium quality olive oil, well worth the money. It is yellow, not green, as good olive oil should be) Spectrum Organic Brown Rice Vinegar Stonewall Kitchen Lemongrass Ginger Oil (1-800-207-5267) Trader Joe's Organic Extra Virgin Olive Oil Wild Thymes Cranberry Ginger and Raspberry Balsamic Vinegar (1-800-724-2877) (Great!)

STORE:	PRODUCT RATING:
LIST PRODUCTS BELOW:	
1.	
2.	
3.	
4.	
5.	
6.	
7.	
8.	
9.	
10.	
11.	
12.	
13.	
14.	
15.	
16.	
17.	
18.	
19.	
20.	
21.	
22.	
23.	
24.	
25.	
26.	
27.	
28.	

STORE:	PRODUCT
LIST PRODUCTS BELOW:	**RATING:**
1.	
2.	
3.	
4.	
5.	
6.	
7.	
8.	
9.	
10.	
11.	
12.	
13.	
14.	
15.	
16.	
17.	
18.	
19.	
20.	
21.	
22.	
23.	
24.	
25.	
26.	
27.	
28.	

STORE:	PRODUCT RATING:
LIST PRODUCTS BELOW:	
1.	
2.	
3.	
4.	
5.	
6.	
7.	
8.	
9.	
10.	
11.	
12.	
13.	
14.	
15.	
16.	
17.	
18.	
19.	
20.	
21.	
22.	
23.	
24.	
25.	
26.	
27.	
28.	

KITCHEN TIPS
COOKING TECHNIQUES

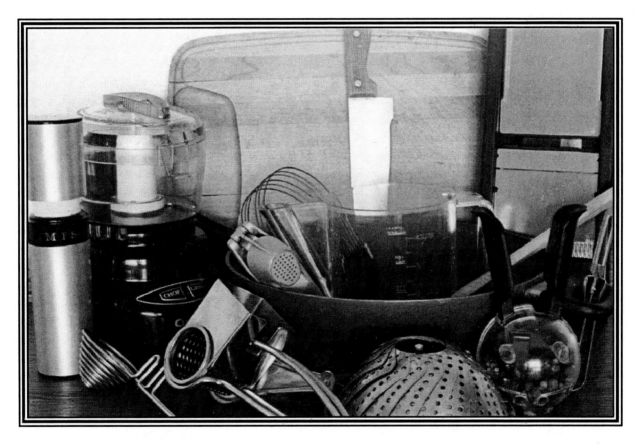

Helpful kitchen gadgets from left to right: oil pump sprayer, small food processor, garlic press, fat separator, mandolin (slicer), vegetable peeler, pepper ball, vegetable steamer, cheese grater, egg separator

KITCHEN TIPS

Eggs:
1. When making deviled eggs, before slicing the egg, dip the knife in water so the yolk won't stick to knife.
2. The white of an egg is easiest to beat when it is at room temperature (about a ½ hour)
3. Add 1 teaspoon cream of tartar to each cup of egg whites to make stiff.
4. A really fresh egg will float and a stale one will sink.
5. If you want to know if an egg is fresh or hardboiled, spin it. If it wobbles, it is raw. It will spin easily if it is boiled.
6. You can use 2 egg whites instead of a whole egg in a recipe in order to get all of the protein and none of the fat.
7. When using several eggs, always crack them separately into a cup and then pour one by one into your mixing bowl so you don't get pieces of shell into your other ingredients or yellow in your whites or vice versa.
8. When recipe calls for adding raw eggs to hot mixture, always begin by adding a small amount of hot mixture to the beaten eggs slowly to avoid curdling.

Baking:
1. To get an accurate measurement when using single cups (1/8, 1/4, ½, 1 cup) or tablespoons or teaspoons, spoon flour etc. into your cup or tablespoon and level with knife.
2. White sugar, brown sugar, and honey may be interchanged (substituted) equally. Because honey is a liquid, if it is exchanged for the dry measurement of sugar, decrease another liquid ingredient in the recipe by the same amount as the honey.
3. If a recipe calls for 1 tablespoon of cornstarch, use 2 tablespoons flour
4. 1 teaspoon of baking powder can be substituted by 1/4 teaspoon baking soda plus ½ teaspoon cream of tartar.
5. Use unbleached white flour or better still, wheat flour.
6. Run a knife around the edges of a cheesecake when it comes out of the oven to prevent cracks from forming.
7. Bake a double crusted pie with two strands of spaghetti sticking up in it to absorb any excess liquid. Let the top part of the spaghetti stick up a few inches. When the pie bakes, if there is any excess liquid inside of it, the liquid will climb up the spaghetti instead of pouring out the sides or the top.
8. Spray measuring spoons or cups with a little oil before measuring sticky ingredients, such as honey, so it will slide right off.
9. Honey will crystallize over time. It doesn't hurt the honey. Just put the container in warm water until the crystals are gone. Don't refrigerate honey, store at room temperature
10. To eliminate fat from a recipe, substitute an equal measurement of natural applesauce in place of oil, butter, sugar or molasses.

Baking Bread:
The reasons for bread not rising are:
1. The liquids were too warm
2. All-purpose flour was used in place of bread flour
3. Rye breads often are small loaves. Rye flour gluten does not become elastic when it is kneaded, nor does it support the structure of the bread. Using an egg even when it is not listed as an ingredient will strengthen the structure and give a better volume. Remember to decrease the total liquid amount by 1/4 cup for each egg added.

4.   There is not enough sugar in the recipe. When liquid is decreased in hot humid weather, sugar may need to be increased. A general rule is to use one tablespoon of sugar with each cup of flour.

5.   Too much sugar will also cause a loaf not to rise. This may happen when fruit is in the recipe. It can be corrected by decreasing the sugar.

6.   A teaspoon of lemon juice will act as a dough conditioner and help to increase the volume of the loaf.

Reasons for bread collapsing:

1.   Liquid temperatures are too warm. Although 80 degrees is the recommended temperature, during very hot and humid conditions the liquid temperature could be cooler.

2.   Too much liquid. Moisture levels of flours vary depending on the relative humidity. Too correct: for 2 cups flour use ½ to 1/4 cup liquid and for 3 cups flour use 1 to 1 1/4 cups liquid. If after reducing liquids, the bread machine labors or hesitates as it is kneading or if the dough forms two balls instead of one, add one tablespoon of liquid at a time until the bread machine is functioning smoothly.

3.   Sometimes the amount of salt will have to be increased. Salt acts like a policeman to yeast making it grow slow and steady.

4.   The correct temperature for yeast is 75 degrees and 85 degrees.

Whenever you make homemade bread or buy "good" bread, finely shred the leftover bread and put in zipper bag and freeze for stuffing.

Yeast: To test yeast to see if it is active, dissolve 1 teaspoon of granulated sugar in ½ cup warm water in a 1 cup measuring cup (110-115 F). Sprinkle 1 packet of yeast (2 1/4 teaspoons) slowly over the surface. Stir the yeast, then set a timer for 10 minutes. In 3 or 4 minutes it will have absorbed enough liquid to activate and will start rising to the surface. If at the end of 10 minutes the yeast has multiplied to the 1 cup mark and has a rounded crown, it is very active. The yeast mixture may be used in your dough. Remember to deduct ½ cup of liquid from the total liquid used in the recipe.

To use Quick Rise Yeast, use ½ teaspoon yeast for each cup of flour in the recipe.
Opened packages of yeast deteriorate very quickly, therefore store in airtight container and refrigerate.

Cooking:

1.   Defatting broths, stews and gravies: Plan to prepare the food several hours or a day ahead and chill it. Then, before reheating the food, simply lift off the hardened fat that has formed on the surface. When there is no time to chill the liquid, float a few ice cubes on the surface of the warm liquid to harden the fat, then remove with a spoon. Another way to remove fat from small amounts of liquid (2 cups or less) is to use a specially designed measuring cup that has the spout at the bottom. Since fat rises to the top, you can pour off the fat-free liquid and leave the fat layer in the measuring cup, discard, and repeat for the rest of the broth.

2.   Never put a cover on anything that is cooked in milk unless you want to spend hours cleaning up the stove when it boils over.

3.   Put a tablespoon of butter in the water when cooking rice, dried beans, pasta to keep it from boiling over. Always run cold water over it when done to get out the starch.

4.   Add a little oil when sauteeing with butter, it will keep the butter from burning.

5.   Browned butter brings out it's flavor, so not as much is needed when adding to vegetables.

6.   Grate cheese as you need it. It will turn moldy if you grate it and store it that way.

7.   Fresh mozzarella cheese is very soft so it is hard to grate. It can be frozen, placed in a plastic bag and placed in water for a few minutes and then grated.
8.   Reheat leftovers in foil in a slow oven.
9.   Stick a wooden spoon handle into hot oil. If it bubbles around the handle, it is ready.

Meat and Fish:
1.   Buy your meat from the butcher, not pre-packaged which may have additives. The meat in the case that is the store brand most often will not have additives, ask the butcher. Filet or sirloin has less fat. Prime rib has the most. The light meat in poultry has the least amount of fat.
2.   Soak fish, shrimp and chicken in milk half an hour to an hour before cooking to remove iodine taste and fishy smell from fish and makes chicken very tender.

Freezing Foods:
1.   To freeze pre-cooked foods, place in freezer with the temperature set at zero degrees as soon as possible after preparing it. Food that is very hot should be cooled first so it won't raise the temperature in the freezer and possibly cause other foods to start thawing. Freeze food in an airtight, moisture resistant package to retain best quality and avoid freezer burn. The best way to do this is to purchase a vacuum seal bag machine but if you can't do that, use combination wrapping. For example, wrap first in a zipper plastic freezer bag and then in heavy duty foil. If you're using a rigid plastic container, first line it with a freezer bag to make it airtight. Divide food into small, serving size portions, if possible. For best quality, use meat within 3 months. Be sure to date packages and put the quantity.
2.   Buy chicken breasts in quantity when they are on sale, wrap each breast individually (sandwich zipper bags) and freeze. They defrost quickly and cut more easily, for stir fry, etc, when they are partially frozen.
3.   Freeze small amounts of leftover sauces or chicken broth in ice cube trays. Pop cubes out after freezing and place cubes in zipper bags. Measure liquid so you'll know how much is in a cube and label the bag as to how much is there.

Miscellaneous:
1.   To clean aluminum pots when they are stained dark, merely boil with a little cream of tartar or vinegar.
2   Lime deposits on tea pots: add vinegar to cover bottom, 1 tablespoon salt. Bring to a boil, remove from heat and scrub.
3.   Clogged drains: (grease) pour 1 cup salt and 1 cup baking soda into drain followed by a kettle of boiling water.
4   Baking powder will remove tea or coffee stains from china pots or cups
5.   Learn where your fuse box and master cut-off switch is and where the gas & water valves are and how to turn them off. Pilot light should be blue, not orange.
7.   Try to use all chemical free cleaning products. There are books available on how to make your own which are much safer, especially with children in the house.

Kitchen Tools:
The right kitchen tools make cooking easier, such as: a good blender or food processor, food chopper, garlic press, good stick free cookware, sharp knives, fat separator, vegetable steamer, pump bottle for oil (use regular olive or canola oil instead of store bought oil spray which contain many additives). Also neat to have: a bread maker, mandolin (slicer), crepe maker, rotisserie, omelet pan, egg poacher, wok, tortilla maker, pasta maker, food bag sealer.

COOKING TECHNIQUES:

Roasted Garlic:
Roasted garlic has an almost sweet flavor and all the harshness and bite seems to disappear. It's great to use on garlic bread or in different recipes.
Remove the papery outer layer. Cut off ends. Place garlic in a small baking dish or foil. Dot them with butter and add enough water so that they are resting in a little liquid. Cover with foil and bake in a 350 degree oven for 45 minutes to one hour. Uncover and bake for 10 minutes more. Mash with fork.

Making a Roux:
A roux is a mixture of flour and butter that is the thickening agent that is used in sauces, soups, stews. This method eliminates the raw taste of flour. To make a roux, follow the proportions of butter to flour in your recipe. Melt the butter over a low heat and then blend in the flour over a period of 3 to 5 minutes. The longer the flour cooks, the more it will color. You must keep the heat low and stir constantly, do not let it burn.

How to Hard Boil an Egg Perfectly:
Put 2 to 12 eggs in a saucepan and cover with cold water at least an inch above eggs. Cover and bring to a boil. Remove from heat, keep covered, and let stand for 15 minutes. Run cold water over and peel immediately.

Dried Tomatoes:
Cut 12 meaty plum tomatoes in half lengthwise. Toss with 1/4 cup olive oil and season with coarse salt, freshly ground pepper and coarsely chopped fresh herbs such as oregano, basil, marjoram, flat-leaf parsley. Line a baking sheet with parchment paper or use a non-aluminum baking dish. Place tomatoes cut side up on baking sheet. Bake in a 275 degree oven until shriveled but still moist about 1 ½ hours to 2 ½ hours. Keep refrigerated in an airtight container for up to one week.

Roasting Peppers:
Roasting red, yellow, green and chile peppers is so easy and makes them taste so much better! Cut in half, cut off stem, remove seeds and membrane. Push with the palm of your hand so it lays flat. Roast on grill on low, closed until black. Place in brown bag for 15 minutes. When you take it out, it should peel easily. You can also do in oven, place on foil or cookie sheet, broil until black with the rack up on highest level. It takes approximately 7-10 minutes but check often. Put in brown bag or zipper bag for 15 minutes. Skin will peel off easily. Dice as needed. Do several at a time and use for your recipe and an omelet the next morning.

Clarified Butter:
Place 1 stick of butter in a small saucepan and melt over low heat. Remove from heat and allow milk solids to sink to bottom. Skim any foam from surface and then carefully pour off golden clarified butter, leaving solids behind.

Clarifying Stock:
This is a method used when you want a clear soup. Clarifying removes solid flecks that are too small to be strained out with cheesecloth, but which will muddy a soup's appearance. To clarify, stir together 1/4 cup of cold water, 1 egg white and 1 egg shell, crushed. Add to strained stock; bring to boiling. Remove from heat and let stand 5 minutes. Strain again through a sieve lined with cheesecloth.

SELECTING FRESH FRUITS AND VEGETABLES

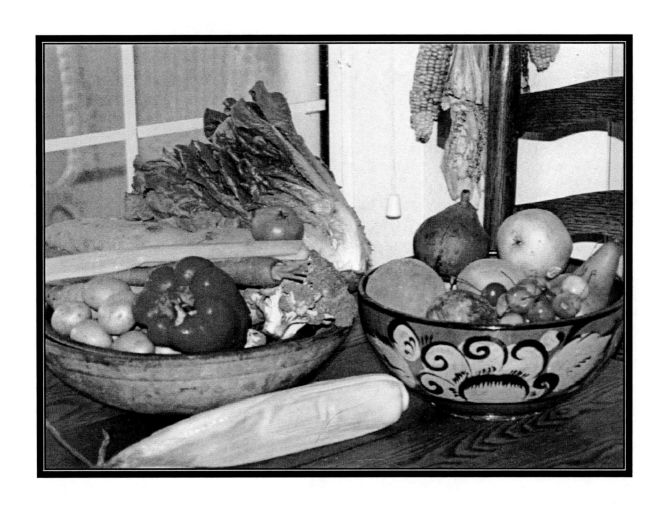

TIPS ON SELECTING FRESH FRUITS & VEGETABLES

Artichoke: Tight leaves, not blooming, may have white or bronze colored blistering caused by frost which does not hurt them. **Avoid:** extremely hard outer leaves opening or spreading.

Asparagus: Fresh spears stand straight, tips tightly closed. Bright green spears with white ends retain moisture better than all green spears. Purple tinged asparagus, grown in cool weather, tends to be sweet; while asparagus grown underground is sharp tasting. Refrigerate with damp paper towel around its ends, then sealed in a plastic bag, asparagus keeps about a week. If ridges form on stems (a sign of age), soak in ice water. **Avoid:** limp or stalks that are too thin.

Beans, green: Fresh, clean, tender, crisp, well shaped. Thin beans are the most tender, can be short or long, smooth skin. Wash before refrigerating but do not snap off ends before storing. Will keep several days in plastic container but best when used immediately. **Avoid:** tough, discolored, soft, wrinkled, lumpy sections along length.

Broccoli: Should be dark green to almost blue on the flower end and be tightly budded. **Avoid:** flower end that is soft enough to easily part with your finger tips and limp or yellow crown.

Cabbage: Semi solid, well rounded, heavy in relation to size, even green coloring, fairly thick leaves will be more tender and juicy. **Avoid:** ones that have thin, wilted leaves or light colored & very solid. Oblong or cracked.

Corn: Full, evenly formed and filled ears, straight rows, fresh looking and bright green husks, silk ends free of decay or worm damage. Kernels bright and shiny. Pull back husk and poke one of the kernels at the tip of the silk end with a fingernail. If juice squirts out and is only slightly cloudy, the corn is fresh. If juice is thick or non-existent, the corn is old. **Avoid:** shriveled, burned looking husks or dark colored slime in the tassel, large kernels or those with dark yellow and dents, wrinkled kernels with no juice in them, all indications of old corn. Also, undeveloped kernels lacking good color (except in white corn). Short or crooked ears that are not filled almost to the tip with kernels.

Carrots: Try to buy carrots with the green tops still on, this guarantees freshness and sweetness. Refrigerate carrots in plastic bags (with moisture draining green tops removed) far from fruits. Ethylene gas makes carrots bitter tasting.

Cauliflower: Choose cauliflower uniform in color, no spots, white, its florets tightly packed together, its jacket leaves dark green and crisp. Refrigerate the cauliflower head in its cellophane wrapper or a plastic bag.

Celery: Even colored, unblemished, smooth skinned leaves, no wilt. Light green tastes best (but not white), scratch butt end, should taste sweet, not bitter. **Avoid:** soft, spreading out, bending, thick veins & rough inside. To revive soft celery, shave small amount from butt end, soak in lukewarm water for ½ hour and refrigerate.

Cucumber: It's ends reveal its age. Old cukes are shriveled, spongy. Keep them in produce drawer of refrigerator, nowhere near the fruits whose ethylene gas hardens a cuke's seeds.

Eggplant: Look for glossy, firm eggplants with smooth, taut skin and a green cap.
Avoid: Large eggplants and those with soft, brown patches may be bitter.

Jicama: Smooth skin free of blemishes, firm and heavy with moisture. Avoid: soft, wrinkled, pock marked, spots of mold. Keep in cool, dry area. Too much moisture will cause mold. Eat raw, in soups, stews, salads. Great substitute for water chestnuts in stir fry.

Peppers: Firm, smooth, solid green. **Avoid:** wrinkles, soft, spots.

Potatoes: Store in a cool, dark, airy place, not in the refrigerator. Chilled, their starch turns to sugar, changing the potato's taste and color.

Red Potatoes: Firm, smooth, bright red, few eyes. Those few eyes should be shallow.
Avoid: soft, wrinkled, cuts in skin, green tinted.

Sweet Potatoes: Tan to light rose. **Avoid:** soft, wrinkled, cuts in skin, white streaks or spots on the inside, will be pithy. The same goes for yams.

Romaine: Large, moderately firm heads, thick leaves, medium dark green nearly white ribs. Even shaped heads, loose leaves. Scratch & smell stalk, should smell sweet, not bitter.

Spinach: Broad, thick, crisp dark leaves, stems unblemished, free of mud. **Avoid:** thin, limp, pale green or yellow. When washing add small amount of salt to cold water, swish, put in colander, rinse, drain and dry.

Squash: Soft shell "summer" squashes, such as zucchini and yellow squash, are harvested young, have edible thin skins and soft seeds. The tastiest are small, the freshest are firm with smooth, shiny skin. Refrigerate and use within 3 to 5 days. Hard shell "winter" squashes, like acorn, butternut and pumpkin, mature on the vine. Skins and seeds are tough. Buy them hard and heavy for their size with a dull finish.

Tomatoes: Never buy a chilled tomato: however red it gets, it will be mushy and tasteless. Pink-orange tomatoes redden in 4 days. Fully ripe tomatoes are deep reddish orange, smell tomatoey and yield to light pressure. They keep at room temperature a day or so. If you must refrigerate them do so only briefly.

Zucchini: Firm, smooth, small, shiny, dark green. Large ones are less tender.
Avoid: wrinkled, blemished or dull.

Apples: Test firmness of apples by holding them in the palm of your hand, do not push with thumb. It should feel solid and heavy, not soft and light. If apple skin wrinkles when you rub your thumb across it, its been in cold storage too long or not kept cold enough.

Red Delicious - not good for baking
Rome - best for baking
Granny Smith - good for baking
Golden Delicious - good for baking and applesauce

Apricot: Fairly firm, dark yellow or yellow orange, they are quite fragile, handle with care and keep at room temperature until ripe.

Blackberry: Firm, good color. Very perishable, handle with care. Keep dry and cool in refrigerator. Do not wash until ready to use.

Blueberries: Firm, plump, uniform in size. Deep purple to nearly black, silver to white frost on the skin, dry and free from leaves. **Avoid:** dull, soft, leaking juice.

Cherries: Large, firm, deep even red coloring. **Avoid:** soft, wrinkled, leaking, sticky.

Cranberry: A good cranberry will bounce. Buy hard, bright, light to dark red berries. Sealed in a plastic bag, they will keep refrigerated for a month, frozen up to a year.

Pears: Store at room temperature until ripe, then refrigerate. You can ripen by placing in a sealed bag with a ripe banana. Should be yellow/green, some red blush, should yield to gentle pressure at stem end. **Avoid:** scars or bruises, too much yellow.

Peach: Large, firm but slightly soft, yellowish background, may have red blush, smell sweet. Avoid: small, hard or too soft, wrinkled, green background will not ripen well.

Plum: Fairly firm to slightly soft smooth skin. Deep even purple color. **Avoid:** extremely hard, wrinkled, punctured or rough skin, or brown discolorations.

Raspberry: Firm, plump, dry. **Avoid:** too firm, green or still attached to stem, mashed or leaking.

Strawberry: Firm but not rock hard, evenly shaped, medium to large, color even and bright red. **Avoid:** wrinkled, soft, spotted with mold, leaking. Berries with more than a touch of green or white around the caps do not ripen well after they are picked.

Watermelon: The ground based side of a perfect watermelon is yellow. The rest of the rind is smooth, waxy, green with or without stripes. If cut, pick bright, crisp, even colored flesh. When you "thump" it will feel like a vibration. Whole melons can stay unrefrigerated for a few days. Once cut, keep covered and cold.

MORE TIPS ON FRUITS AND VEGETABLES

To ripen green fruit: place in a paper bag and store at room temperature until ripe.
If fresh veggies are wilted or blemished, pick off the brown edges, sprinkle with cold water, wrap in a clean towel and refrigerate for an hour or so.

Store tomatoes stems down, never refrigerate them as they lose all of their flavor.
Never refrigerate potatoes, they turn to starch.

To prevent wilting and molding, never wash fruits and vegetables until ready to use. Store in crisper in your refrigerator and use as soon as possible.

To hurry up baked potatoes, boil in salted water for 10 minutes, then place in very hot oven or cut potatoes in half and place them face down on a baking sheet.

To cook corn on a grill, remove silk, put cob back into husk and soak for a half an hour or so. Dry corn and spread on butter, put back in husk. Shred a piece of husk into a thin tie and use to tie husk at top. Make sure corn is covered by husk. Put on grill and turn often. Takes about 20 minutes.

Steam vegetables in as little water as possible to prevent vitamins from leaking into water. Raw, of course, is best for you. If you need to cook vegetables for a longer time (with other ingredients), cut in large pieces to expose fewer surfaces to water and heat. Leave skin on certain fruits and vegetables such as carrots, potatoes, cucumbers, apples, peaches, pears. The skin is an important source of fiber and nutrients. Just scrub well with a vegetable brush under cold running water.

Anything that grows under the ground, start off in cold water: potatoes, carrots, etc.

Anything that grows above the ground, start off in boiling water: peas, greens, beans, etc.

FRESH CORN KERNALS

Kernals cut from fresh ears of corn can add taste and texture to chowders, pasta dishes, and salads. (One medium size ear of corn yields about ½ cup kernals.)

To remove the kernals, place a cutting board on top of a damp towel so it won't slip. Use a large knife to cut the large end of an ear of corn flat. Then hold the ear vertically, with the flat end pressed into the cutting board. Use a sharp knife to cut the kernals from the cob; do not scrape cob.

TIPS ON POTATOES

1. Red and golden skinned potatoes should be taut and shiny
2. Select potatoes uniform in size so they will cook evenly
3. The potatoes skin reveals a great deal about quality and freshness, look for those with no signs of sprouting, shriveling or bruising
4. Extremes of heat and cold damage potatoes. Store them in a dark, airy, cool spot in an open paper bag, not sealed in plastic
5. Don't refrigerate or freeze potatoes. This turns the potato starch into sugar

6. Don't wash potatoes before storing because it speeds the development of decay. Instead, scrub potatoes under running water just before preparing.

7. Once potatoes are peeled or cut, an enzyme causes the flesh to darken. To prevent discoloration, keep cut potatoes submerged in cold water until ready to use

8. When boiling potatoes, start them in cold water to cover. Choose a saucepan that will be only about two thirds full, to avoid boiling over. Once the water comes to a boil, decrease the heat to achieve a steady simmer

9. Classified as a vegetable, a potato provides 45 percent of the daily value for vitamin C, 21 percent of the daily value for potassium, 3 grams of fiber and 100 calories

SPICES, HERBS AND THEIR USES

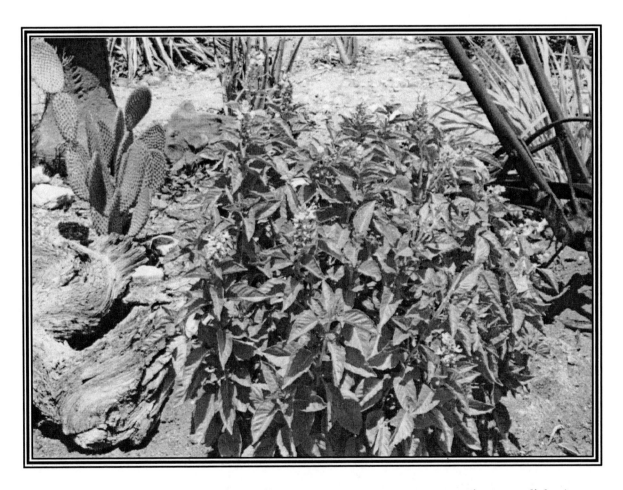

My organically grown sweet basil (very easy to grow, tastes great in many dishes)

ALLSPICE	Resembles cloves and nutmeg, fragrant and pungent taste, used in baking
BAY LEAVES	Seasoning for soups, stews and sauces (spaghetti sauce), use sparingly, can be bitter
CARDAMOM	Sweet flavor, bread, fruit, apple dishes, sweet potatoes, curries
CAYENNE PEPPER	HOT, use sparingly, a little provides a lot of flavor and heat to any dish
CELERY SEED	Enhances celery taste in soups, sauces, salad dressings
CILANTRO	Use in Mexican dishes, Fresh is always best
CINNAMON	Use in sweet and savory foods, desserts
CLOVES	Strong, bitter taste but mellows when cooked with other ingredients, use with cinnamon and nutmeg, desserts
CORIANDER	Has a slight lemon flavor, rub on beef, chicken, pork, fish and lamb, spareribs. Add to chicken soup, use in cakes, cookies, biscuits, apple dishes
CREAM OF TARTER	Use in Angel Cake & meringues (used to stabilize beaten egg whites)
CUMIN	Sweet aroma, somewhat bitter and pungent, use with coriander, cinnamon, chile, crushed pepper and pepper. Use in Mexican cooking, rub on meats and chicken before roasting
CURRY	Indian dishes
DILL	Use in seafood and vegetable dishes. Great with carrots
DRY MUSTARD	Ground seed of the mustard (spicy) use to make homemade mustard or vegetables, meat, eggs and poultry
GARLIC POWDER	A little goes a long way. Meats, soups, sauces, pasta dishes, in butter for bread
GINGER	Use in cakes, cookies, gingerbread, fruit, puddings, oriental dishes, lamb, pork, beef, chicken or veal, salad dressing. Fresh ginger is great
LEMON PEPPER BLEND	Black pepper, lemon peel, coriander, onion, thyme, lemon oil.Use in vegetables, marinades when grilling meat, poultry and fish, salads, dips
MARGORAM	Similar to oregano. Use in soups, sauces, roasts (lamb). Mix with rosemary and thyme
MINT	Good with fruit, lamb, roast. Fresh is best.
NUTMEG	Great in lots of baked goods. Whole fresh nutmeg is always best.
ONION POWDER	1 tablespoon=1 onion
OREGANO	Use with all Italian dishes. Fresh is always best.
PAPRIKA	Sauces, deviled eggs, chicken, beef, pork, Mexican dishes
PARSLEY	Salads, soups, vegetables, potatoes, casseroles, pork, fish, egg dishes
POULTRY SEAS.	basil, rosemary, sage, marjoram, thyme, oregano (stuffing, eggs, fish, poultry
ROSEMARY	Potatoes, bread. Fresh is always best
SAGE	Use with Poultry and all stuffing, soups, sauces, carrots, eggplant, peas,tomatoes
TARRAGON	Use in soup, spinach, squash, corn, cauliflower, potato, tuna, chicken, egg, pasta salad, sauces, fish, salads, Bearnaise sauce
THYME	Spicy. Use in creole dishes and stuffing, rub on game birds or roasts
TUMERIC	Peppery and pungent. In the ginger family. Use in Indian dishes, vegetable dishes

VANILLA BEAN	Pick beans that are tender and near black. Desserts.
WHITE PEPPER	A general seasoning. Good used on fish, mashed potatoes, white sauce, salad dressing, cheese sauce, soup, eggs, omelets, use in a shaker on the table (a little milder than black pepper)

Read labels on spices to make sure they don't contain additives. Most Paprika does. I use Szeged Hungarian paprika. A lot of spices may contain MSG. Spice Hunter is a very good natural brand that does not.

Dried spices and herbs are only good for about six months at the most. If they don't have a strong smell, they won't add to the flavor of your food. When you buy spices, write the date on the jar. Buy only small quantities at a time. The best way to buy spices is in the whole form. Use a spice grinder or coffee grinder used just for spices and grind as needed. Wipe out with a paper towel after use. Don't wash. Most grocery stores carry fresh herbs, if you can't grow your own. You may freeze any leftover, just make sure they are dry and loosely put in freezer bag.

Fresh ginger is great to have on hand. Since you don't use much at a time and it goes bad quickly, store in a zipper bag in the freezer. Cut off piece as needed, immerse in hot water and the skin comes off and it is ready to chop.

Remove small leaves from fresh herbs like thyme and marjoram by pinching the tip of the herb stem and sliding it in the opposite direction of the leaf growth to the base. The delicate tips can be used along with leaves.

The stems in fresh cilantro have a lot of flavor, so chop them along with the leaves.

FRESH HORSERADISH ROOT

Horseradish is a low calorie, natural condiment that adds a distinctive, pungent flavor to foods. It is commonly used as a relish with meats and shellfish or as a tangy seasoning in sauces served with these foods. Add prepared horseradish (directions at the bottom of page) to taste, to any of the following: egg dishes (such as deviled eggs, egg salad, omelets, scrambled eggs), cream cheese, mayonnaise, or butter for use as a spread on sandwiches, sour cream or creme fraiche along with salt, pepper, paprika, cayenne, etc. for dip, put in coleslaw, potato salad, barbeque sauce, fondue, salad dressings, and gravies, for extra zing. Add to "good" ketchup for a quick and easy shrimp sauce. Some cooks use it generously to give a hot taste to food, others find that a small amount of horseradish is sufficient to impart a subtle, delightful flavor that turns an ordinary dish into an extra special one.

The name horseradish has nothing to do with horses and it is not a radish. It's actually a member of the mustard family. The name may have come from an English adaptation of its German name.

The sharp flavor and penetrating smell of horseradish become apparent when the root is grated or ground. This is because the root contains highly volatile oils that are released by enzyme activity when the root cells are crushed. If exposed to air or stored improperly, horseradish loses its pungency rapidly after grinding.

To keep prepared horseradish at its flavorful best, store it in a tightly covered jar in the refrigerator or in the freezer. It will keep its good quality for about 4 to 6 weeks in the refrigerator and for six months or longer in the freezer. I buy a fresh root, in the produce section of the store. Make sure it is clean, firm and free from cuts and deep blemishes. The whiter the root, the fresher it is. Immediately place it in an airtight bag, place in the freezer and cut off a piece as needed, place back in freezer.

Grind fresh horseradish in a well ventilated room. The fumes from grinding are potent, a whiff may be stronger than you expect. Wash and peel the root and dice it into small cubes. Place the cubes into a blender or food processor. Process a small amount at a time. Add cold water to cover the blades and put cover on blender or food processor. Process until right consistency and add more water if needed. For each cup of horseradish, add 2 to 3 tablespoons of white vinegar and ½ teaspoon of salt. A tablespoon of sugar can be substituted for the salt. The time at which you add the vinegar is important. Vinegar stops the enzymatic action in the ground product and stabilizes the degree of hotness. If you prefer horseradish that is not too hot, add the vinegar immediately. If you like it as hot as it can be, wait three minutes before adding the vinegar. Store in jar with tight fitting lid, date, and store in the refrigerator for 4 weeks.

FOOD SAFETY

1. Scrub hands with soap and water for at least 20 seconds before, during, and after food preparation. For picnics, take along disposable, antibacterial, moist towelettes.

2. Clean all surfaces before and after food preparation with hot, soapy water or with a sanitizing solution of 1 tablespoon chlorine bleach in a bucket of water.

3. Clean sponges often and, when possible, use disposable towels instead of cloth to clean kitchen messes. According to a University study, the typical damp household sponge houses 700 million microorganisms. Soak used sponges in a bleach solution of 3/4 cup bleach per 1 gallon of water.

4. Keep raw meat, fish, and poultry and the knives and cutting boards used to prepare them, away from other foods. Cross contamination, where harmful bacteria from raw food is passed on to safe food, is responsible for more than one third of food borne illnesses.

5. Eggs have been known to carry the harmful salmonella bacteria. To reduce the risk of infection, use only fresh, clean, refrigerated eggs that are free of any cracks. If a recipe calls for room temperature eggs, place the uncracked eggs in a bowl of hot water for 5 minutes so they can lose their chill.

6. Wash all cutting boards and utensils in hot, soapy water immediately after each use. You can also purchase inexpensive, disposable cutting boards.

7. Keep hot foods hot (above 140 degrees) and cold foods cold (below 40 degrees). Germs thrive between 40 degrees and 140 degrees. Under ideal conditions, one bacterium can morph into 17 million in just eight hours. A thermometer is one of your best weapons in the fight against food borne illnesses.

8. Cook red meat, ground meat, ground poultry and fish to 160 degrees and poultry to 180 degrees. Reheat cooked foods to 180 degrees.

9. Keep your freezer set at 0 degrees or colder and the refrigerator at 32 -37 degrees.

10. When shopping, purchase perishables and frozen foods last. If you can't make it home within 30 minutes of shopping, store food in an ice filled cooler.

11. Defrost frozen food overnight in the refrigerator or in cold water, changing the water every 30 minutes. Food defrosted in the microwave oven should be cooked right away.

12. Pack for picnics right before you leave, using plenty of ice. Store drinks in a separate cooler to avoid opening the food cooler constantly. Keep coolers in a shady cool place with the lids tightly closed. Add more ice as it melts.

PREVIEW TO RECIPES

1.   Use your menu planners so you avoid needless trips to the store.

2.   Read the recipe all the way through before starting to cook. I find it very helpful to gather ingredients and measure seasonings into a small bowl before starting.

3.   Preheat oven for 10 minutes on all recipes.

4.   Always use a meat thermometer to make sure your meat and poultry is throughly cooked.

5.   I have included a Rub recipe, a combination of spices and herbs, at the beginning of the Chicken, Beef, Pork and Fish chapters. Rubs are a great way to add flavor without fat. There are a lot of good rubs on the market such as Spice Hunter which are all natural, but they are so easy to make. When applied to meats that are slow cooked, rubs soak up the juices and form a tasty crust. To use rubs, first wash and dry the food. You can lightly oil the surface to help the rub stick and to keep the meat moist. Let stand 30 minutes or even over night to let the spices permeate. When making your own combinations use equal parts of spices and salt and pepper to taste. You can also add a little brown or white sugar. A rub should enhance, not overpower the flavor of meat. I like to have these rubs made in advance to cut down on preparation time. They are used in several recipes. Also good to have on hand: mayonnaise, mustard, and frozen chicken stock all of which can be made from recipes in this book.

6.   Make sure meat and poultry are additive free. Even when buying from the butcher ask if anything has been added.

7.   It's always best to use fresh herbs, vegetables and fruits whenever possible. Organic is always the best choice. Growing your own herbs is very easy, but if you can't do that, a lot of grocery stores carry fresh. Freeze any leftover but make sure they are dry and pack lightly. If you have to use dried, half the amount. For example one tablespoon dried or two tablespoons fresh.

8.   A lot of recipes call for dried onion flakes. Fresh onions are a big trigger for a lot of people so I just stick to using the dried. They really taste great and you don't have the tearing problem of fresh onions! Of course, make sure the brand you use are just onions and nothing else added.

9.   Red, yellow, and green peppers and green chilies are used a lot in the recipes. You don't have to roast them, but I think they have a lot more flavor when you do. Look in the Kitchen Techniques section of the book, page 22, for how to roast them.

10.   Using coarse salt or sea salt and freshly ground pepper add a lot of flavor. A pepper mixture of pink, green and black is especially nice. The seasonings in the recipes are to my taste, you may want to use less salt or change seasonings to your liking.

11. Fresh mozzarella cheese is sometimes hard to find, so when I do find it, I freeze it. It is the only cheese I know of that really freezes quite well. Take it out of the freezer, put it in a sealed plastic bag, put it in a little warm water for a few minutes and then grate it. You can actually grate it after it has been frozen and semi thawed. If it is not frozen, you have to cut it up because it is so soft.

12. Farmer cheese is used in some of the recipes. There are two kinds of farmer cheese, one hard and one soft. The one used almost exclusively in this book is the solid kind. The friendship farmer is the soft kind, almost like ricotta. The only recipe using friendship farmer is the Blintze recipe.

13. Unsalted butter is best to use because the amount of salt in salted butter varies from brand to brand and therefore is very difficult to adjust the amount of salt in a recipe.

14. The healthiest oils to use are olive and canola. Always use the best extra virgin olive oil that you can find. It should be golden yellow, not green. Extra virgin guarantees that the oil has been cold pressed from freshly harvested olives and does not contain chemicals and provides the best flavor.

15. I mention a "Silpat" in several recipes. It is a wonderful cookie sheet liner that eliminates having to oil the pan. You can find it in good kitchen stores and some have other brands that are just as good.

16. Creme fraiche and sour cream are interchangeable. Creme fraiche tends to be creamier and milder than sour cream. Most cream products have additives, so when shopping read the labels of both and find a product such as Daisy brand Sour Cream or Vermont Butter and Cheese Company Creme Fraiche.

17. Because whole grain products are much healthier than white, always try to use brown rice, wheat pasta, natural sugar (which is tan), wheat bread or if you use white flour, make sure it is unbleached.

18. I didn't indicate servings on most recipes because appetites vary. Double or half the recipe accordingly.

19. In some of the recipes I suggest brands, however any additive free brand is fine.

20. Remember...some of these recipes are not low fat, low calorie. Unfortunately, low fat products have a lot of "bad" ingredients in them that seem to trigger headaches. The key to not gaining weight is moderation, small portions, exercise and don't eat the higher calorie meals every day. Alternate with the lesser calorie ones. Also, use less cheese, butter and oil if you are worried about fat. Eat a lot of vegetables and fruits, and use and make whole grain food instead of white (rice, bread, pasta).

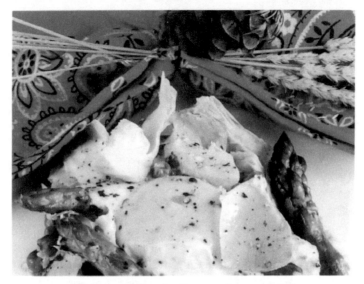

Tony and Fran's Casserole, page 97
Place setting courtesy of Tony and Fran Meredith-Piccione, Columbia River Gorge, WA

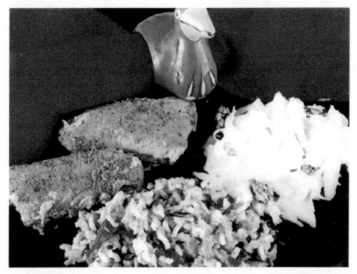

Lori's Spicy Sweet Pepper Rice, page 91, Cole Slaw, page 110, Pork Loin Ribs, page 60
Place setting courtesy of Lori Bentley Law and Brian Law

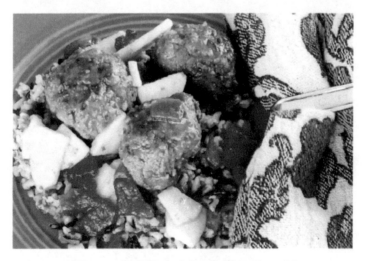

Sweet and Sour Meatballs, page 49
My father, Charles Meredith's napkin ring

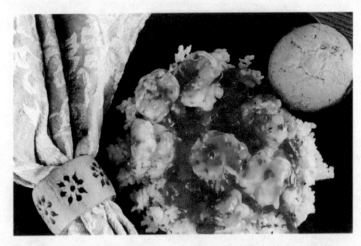

Roger's Spicy Shrimp and Sauce, page 70, Cornmeal Muffin, page 123
Place setting courtesy of Kimberley, James and Jordan Davis

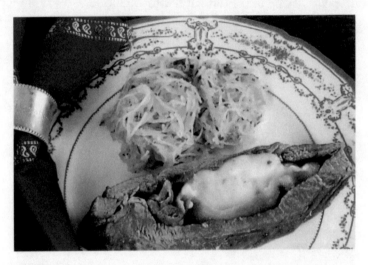

Chile Stuffed Flank Steak, page 53, Spaghetti Squash, page 104
My grandmother, Dorothy Danforth Jewett's napkin ring and china

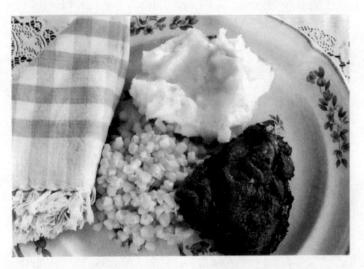

Fried Chicken, page 43, Mashed Potatoes, page 95, Creamed Corn, page 103
Place setting courtesy of Jan, Wayne, Casey, Kayla and Megan Bentley

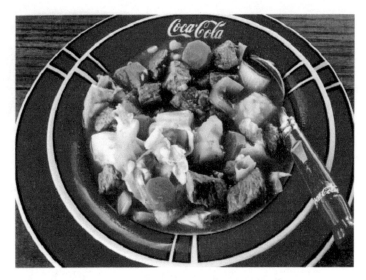

Vegetable Beef Soup, page 115
Place setting courtesy of Gail and Dennis Eastin

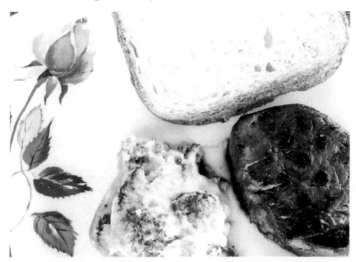

Broccoli Casserole, page 98, Honey Oatmeal Bread, page 120, grilled filet mignon
Plate courtesy of Kristy and Neil Erekson

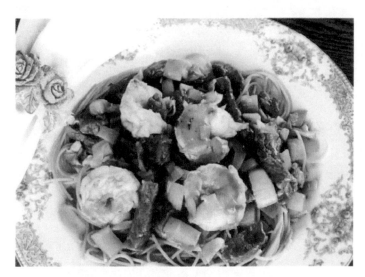

Steak and Shrimp Stir Fry, page 86
Place setting courtesy of Vivian and Greg Belliston and Bertha Walters

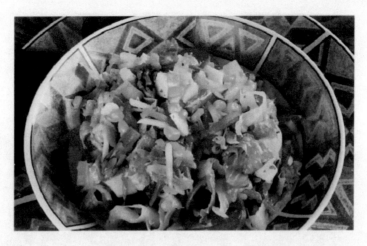

Chopped Salad #2, page 109
Place setting courtesy of Deana and Bob Dufala

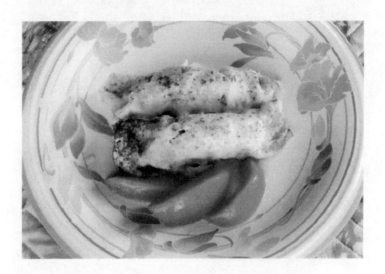

Chicken and Broccoli Crepes, page 38
Place setting courtesy of Barb and Bob Merow

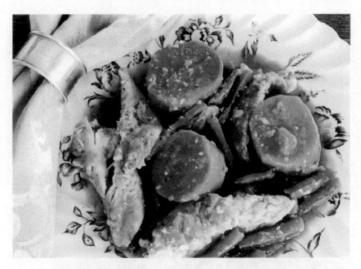

Mom's One Pan Chicken Dish, page 44
Place setting courtesy of Kathie and Jerry Quater

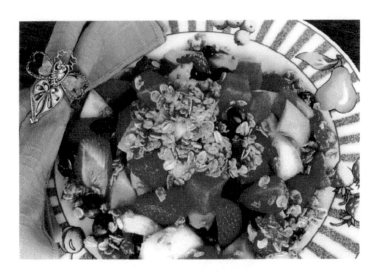

Fruit Salad (without dressing) page 113, Granola, page 157
Angel given to my Mom for her 80th birthday from my dear friend of 44 years, Lynne Schapeler

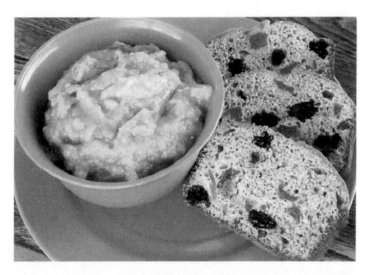

Gramp's Applesauce, page 134, Breakfast Bread, page 128
Place setting courtesy of Hazel Yonts

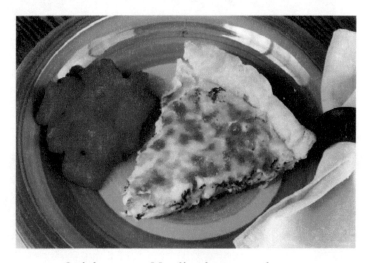

Quiche, page 88, sliced watermelon
Place setting courtesy of Apryl and Brent Erekson

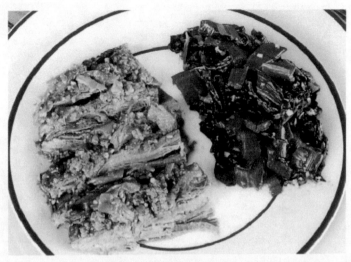

Slow Simmered Flank Steak, page 53, Sauteed Swiss Chard, page 104
Plates courtesy of Vickie and Don Yonts

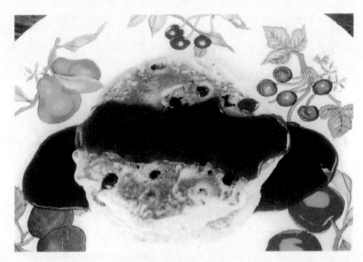

Blueberry Pancakes and Blueberry Syrup, page 128
Plate courtesy of Molly and Larry Troub

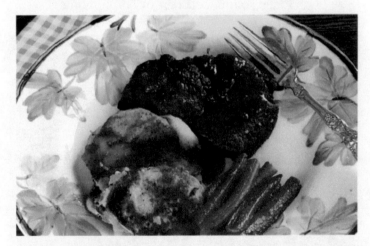

Dried Tomato Meatloaf, page 48, Potato Ring, page 84, Honey Glazed Carrots, page 99
Place setting courtesy of Lura and LaVerne Bertram

CHICKEN DISHES

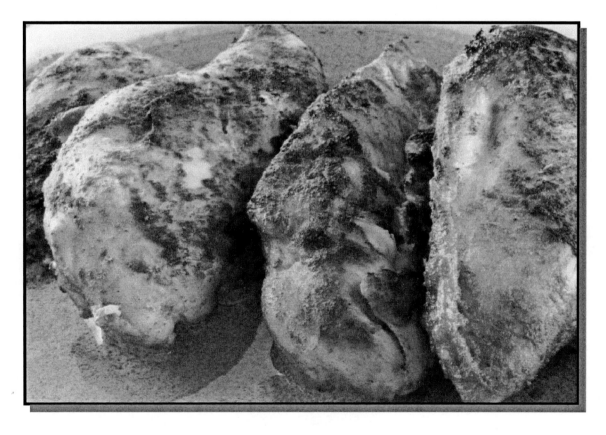

Chicken Paprika, page 36

CHICKEN RUB

This rub is used in several recipes. It is a very good combination of spices for any grilled chicken. Combine spices and put in a jar with a shaker top, sprinkle or rub on both sides of chicken before grilling

1 tablespoon	garlic powder
1 tablespoon	onion powder
1 tablespoon	paprika
1 tablespoon	chili powder
1 tablespoon	cumin
½ teaspoon	salt
½ teaspoon	pepper

Note: Grilling time varies by the cut of the chicken. To minimize dryness, pound the meat to a uniform thickness to allow it to cook evenly. Cook the same parts together. Sear both sides of the raw meat on a hot, open grill to seal in the moisture. Then close the grill. Chicken breasts 1" thick take about 12 to 16 minutes, thinner, flatter ones take about 6-8 minutes, turning 3 times for all. They are done when juices run clear when pierced with the tip of a sharp knife. Don't overcook chicken as it will be tough. Coat the grill surface with oil to prevent sticking. When using marinade, 30 minutes of soaking is enough, unless the recipe specifies a longer time. Discard uncooked leftover marinade.

CHICKEN STOCK

Stock is used in a lot of recipes and is a very good thing to have in the freezer for immediate use

1 large	natural whole chicken (clean out insides and wash)
3 stalks	celery with leaves, washed and cut up
2 medium	carrots, scrubbed and cut up
1 ½ teaspoons	salt
½ teaspoon	pepper
2 tablespoons	dried onion flakes

Put chicken in a large pot and cover with water. Add celery, carrots, salt, pepper and onion. Bring a boil and reduce heat. Cover and simmer for approximately 1 ½ hours or until chicken is done. Lift out chicken and place on platter or cookie sheet. Strain stock through a sieve lined with cheesecloth. Discard vegetables. Chill stock and lift off the solidified fat. Take chicken off bones and discard bones and fat. Freeze or use good meat within a day or two at the most.

Note: It is not necessary to peel or trim vegetables for stock since they will be strained out. Just wash and cut up. Start with cold water to extract the most flavor from meat and vegetables. Simmer stock slowly for best flavor, bubbles should form slowly and burst before reaching the surface. To avoid spills, ladle stock into the strainer rather than pouring it. Avoid over-seasoning stocks for other recipes. Stock may be stored in the refrigerator for a few days or up to 6 months in the freezer. Be sure to label it with the date and amount. If you frequently use stock in small quantities, freeze it in ice cube trays. When frozen, place frozen stock cubes in a plastic bag and return them to the freezer. Measure the volume of a melted cube to determine the exact amount of stock in each cube and label on bag.

Note: When you want a clear soup, clarifying stock removes solid flecks that are too small to be strained out with cheesecloth, but which will muddy a soup's appearance. To clarify, stir together 1/4 cup cold water, 1 egg white, and 1 egg shell, crushed. Add to strained stock, bring to a boil. Remove from heat and let stand 5 minutes. Strain again through a sieve lined with cheesecloth.

ROASTED TURKEY OR CHICKEN WITH STUFFING FOR TWO

4 pound	young turkey or roasting chicken (fresh and additive free)
½ stick (1/4 cup)	butter
3/4 cup	celery
1/4 cup	dried onion flakes
½ teaspoon	salt
1/4 teaspoon	pepper
2 ½ cups	bread crumbs (homemade bread, recipes on pages 120 and 121) or use "good" bread

Melt butter in large pan and add diced celery, onions, salt and pepper. Saute for a minute or two and stir in bread crumbs until well blended. Spoon into washed and dried turkey or chicken. Immediately place in roasting pan. <u>NEVER</u> stuff ahead of time. Place in a 350 degree oven. After an hour and a half, insert a meat thermometer in the center of where the stuffing is. It should read 180 degrees. When the thigh muscle is pierced deeply with a fork, juices should be clear and no longer reddish pink.

Carving Suggestion: Cut band of skin holding drumsticks. Grasp drumstick. Place knife between drumstick/thigh and body of turkey and cut through skin to joint. Remove entire leg by pulling out and back using point of knife to disjoint it. Separate thigh and drumstick at joint. Insert fork in upper wing to steady turkey or chicken. Make a long horizontal cut above wing joint through to body frame. Wing may be disjointed from body, if desired. Beginning halfway up breast, cut thin slice with an even stroke. When knife reaches horizontal cut, slice will fall free. Continue slicing breast meat, starting cut at a higher point each time.

Serving Suggestion: Great served with cranberry sauce. Most people, of course, want gravy. If you don't mind the extra calories, here's a simple recipe for gravy: stir enough flour into pan drippings until very thick and well blended. Over medium heat, add water a half a cup at a time stirring constantly until the consistency you like. Keep stirring for a few minutes until very hot. Add salt to taste. Adjust the amount of stuffing for the weight of the turkey (example: 8 pound turkey, double recipe, and so forth).

TURKEY BREAST AND NEW POTATOES

2 pound	fresh, natural whole turkey breast
2 tablespoons	butter
1 tablespoon	olive oil
2 teaspoons	garlic, minced
2 tablespoons	fresh basil or 1 tablespoon dried basil
3 cups	small new potatoes, cut in half

Place turkey breast in roasting pan. In small frying pan, melt butter and oil. Stir in garlic and basil. Stir until well mixed. Lift up skin on turkey and rub half of mixture underneath skin. Place the rest of mixture in bowl, add potatoes and coat. Set aside.

Place turkey in a 325 degree oven. After an hour, place potatoes around turkey and cook for about another hour or until meat thermometer tests done and potatoes are soft. Stir potatoes once during cooking so they brown on all sides.

BREADED SAUTEED CHICKEN BREASTS

2 large	chicken breasts, boneless, skinless, pounded until thin but be careful not to tear, and seasoned with Rub recipe on page 33
6 tablespoons	olive oil

1/3 cup	unbleached, all purpose flour
1 teaspoon	salt

Mix together on plate

1	egg
1/4 cup	milk

Mix together in shallow bowl

1 cup	finely shredded "good" bread crumbs (best if left on plate overnight or for a few hours to dry)
1 teaspoon	thyme
1 teaspoon	oregano
1 teaspoon	parsley
1 teaspoon	basil
2 tablespoons	finely grated farmer cheese
½ teaspoon	salt

Mix together on plate

Dredge both sides of the pounded, seasoned chicken in flour mixture, then the egg mixture and then the bread crumb mixture and place on plate. Heat the 6 tablespoons olive oil over medium heat and when it is very hot saute the breasts for approximately 3 minutes on each side, high heat, or until brown. Serve immediately with sauce (recipe below).

Sauce:

½ teaspoon	garlic oil
1 teaspoon	garlic, minced
1/8 teaspoon	salt
1 cup	creme fraiche or Daisy sour cream

Heat oil in small frying pan and add garlic. Saute for a minute or so and add salt and creme fraiche until well blended and hot.

Serving Suggestion:　　　Serve with wild or brown rice and corn or carrots.

CHICKEN AND BISCUITS

My husband and kids have always loved this dish! The best way to make it is to boil the chicken the day before, place the stock in a bowl, cover and refrigerate. Pull apart the chicken and throw away the bones, etc. and refrigerate the good pieces. The next day skim the fat off the top of the stock and cut up the chicken

2 cups	cooked chicken, cut up in bite sized pieces
1/4 cup	butter
1/4 cup	flour
1 cup	milk
1 cup	chicken stock
3/4 teaspoon	salt
1/4 teaspoon	pepper
1/4 teaspoon	paprika
1/8 teaspoon	cayenne pepper
1/3 cup	creme fraiche (Vermont Butter & Cheese Co.) or sour cream (Daisy)
1 ½ cups	frozen peas
1	roasted red pepper, diced
1	recipe biscuits (recipe on page 22)

Melt butter over low heat in medium saucepan. Stir in flour until smooth and well blended. Add milk and stock stirring constantly over low heat until thick. Add salt, pepper, paprika, cayenne, and creme fraiche or sour cream. Add peas, cut up chicken and diced red pepper and stir until heated through. Split biscuits and spoon chicken mixture on top.

Note: Freeze the remaining stock (write amount on package) for future use and make chicken salad out of any remaining chicken or freeze for use in another recipe.

CHICKEN PAPRIKA

4	boneless, skinless chicken breasts
	paprika
1 tablespoon	canola or olive oil
1 tablespoon	butter
1 tablespoon	dried onion flakes
1 cup	chicken broth, homemade (recipe on page 33)
½ teaspoon	salt
1/4 teaspoon	pepper
½ cup	creme fraiche (Vermont Butter and Cheese Company) or Daisy sour cream

Place chicken on plate and sprinkle paprika on both sides. Heat oil and butter in skillet and saute chicken until brown on both sides. Take out chicken and quickly saute onion. Add chicken broth, salt, and pepper. Stir up pan drippings until well mixed. Put chicken back in pan with broth. Cover and simmer on low for 30 minutes. Take out chicken and stir in creme fraiche until well blended. Cook and stir for a minute or so until slightly thickened. Pour sauce over chicken and serve immediately.

Serving Suggestion: I like to serve this dish with hot crusty buttered bread and steamed broccoli.

HONEY PEAR CHICKEN AND RICE

Sauce:

1 ½ cups	water
½ cup	honey
1 teaspoon	cardamom
1 cup	pear juice
3	pears, peeled and diced

Combine water, honey, cardamom, and pear juice. Boil down until syrupy. While sauce is simmering, make chicken.

4	chicken breasts, cut in bite size pieces
2 tablespoons	butter
1 tablespoon	fresh chopped basil
1 teaspoon	salt
½ teaspoon	white pepper

Spray a little oil in pan, melt butter and add basil. Add cut up chicken pieces and cook over high heat stirring until well browned and pan is dry. Add ½ cup water to pan and stir up pan drippings over medium high heat until almost all the liquid is gone. Add simmered honey mixture and cook over medium heat until thickened and chicken is coated. Stir in diced pears. Serve over brown or wild rice.

Note: You can also grill chicken, slice into strips and pour sauce over.

OVEN BAKED SPICY CHICKEN

4	boneless, skinless chicken breasts sprinkled with Chicken Rub on page 33
1 ½ cups	milk
1 cup	bread crumbs (recipes on pages 120 and 121 or "good" bread) mixed with ½ teaspoon of Chicken Rub

Place seasoned chicken into a 11" x 8" baking pan. Let sit for 10 minutes. Pour milk over chicken turning to coat. Cover and put in refrigerator for 2 hours, turning chicken occasionally. Remove chicken from dish and discard milk. Dredge chicken in breadcrumbs on both sides and place on oiled baking sheet (or Silpat lined). Bake in a 400 degree oven for 40 minutes (should be browned on top). Do not turn. Serve immediately.

Serving Suggestion: Cut chicken into strips and serve with sweet and sour sauce (recipe on page 49, Sweet and Sour Meatballs sauce or Robbie's Hawaiian Style) for dipping.

CHICKEN AND BROCCOLI CREPES

These crepes are so good and easy to make if you use an inexpensive crepe maker found at most kitchen stores

3 cups	chicken, finely chopped (grill 3 or 4 boneless, skinless chicken breasts rubbed with Chicken Rub, recipe on page 33)
1 cup	broccoli tops, fresh, cut up very small

Crepes:

1 cup	all purpose flour
1 ½ cups	milk
1	egg
1/4 teaspoon	salt

Before you start, tear off 18 sections of wax paper. Place a large plate and the wax paper near where you will be working.

Mix crepe ingredients together until well blended and smooth. If you don't have a crepe maker, you can make them in a 6" non-stick skillet, but it takes a lot of practice. To use the skillet method, rub a little oil with a paper towel on the pan just to lightly coat. Heat skillet until very warm, not hot, to the touch. Remove from heat. Spoon in about 2 tablespoons of batter, lift and tilt skillet to spread batter. Return to medium heat and brown on one side only. Loosen edges carefully with a spatula. Invert pan over waxed paper on plate to remove. Repeat until all the batter is gone placing waxed paper between each crepe. Lightly oil skillet as needed. You'll use about 12 for this recipe. See note below for freezing or using the extras.

Sauce:

2 tablespoons	butter
2 tablespoons	all purpose flour
½ teaspoon	salt
1/4 teaspoon	white pepper
1/8 teaspoon	cayenne
2 ½ cups	milk

Melt butter in saucepan over low heat. Blend in flour until light brown stirring constantly, add salt, pepper, cayenne. Add milk all at once. Stir constantly until thickened and bubbling.

Assemble:

Mix broccoli with chicken and add ½ cup of the sauce. Spoon a packed 1/4 cup of the filling in the center of the unbrowned side of each crepe leaving an inch from each end. Tightly, without tearing, roll up and arrange crepes, seam side down, in a lightly oiled 13" x 9" baking dish. Spoon sauce over each crepe, and sprinkle with a little paprika. Cover with foil and bake in a 350 degree oven for 20 minutes.

Note:	If you have any extra crepes, you can freeze them by stacking them between waxed paper and placing in a large plastic bag or container. You can also use crepes with any fruit for a great dessert.

CREAMY CHICKEN

6	skinless, boneless chicken breasts
½ cup	vinegar (Wild Thymes Cranberry Balsamic)
2 teaspoons	fresh oregano or 1 teaspoon dried oregano
½ teaspoon	salt
½ teaspoon	pepper
1 cup	water
3	garlic cloves, peeled
1/4 cup	milk
1	tablespoon mayonnaise (recipe on page 129)
1/8 teaspoon	salt
1/8 teaspoon	pepper
2	tablespoons minced fresh parsley, or 1 tablespoon dried

Arrange chicken in a 13" x 9" pan. Pour vinegar over chicken, sprinkle with oregano, salt, pepper. Add water. Place whole garlic in pan. Bake in a 350 degree oven for 40 minutes basting occasionally with pan drippings. Remove garlic from pan, put in bowl and mash into paste. Place chicken on platter. Stir milk, mayonnaise, salt, pepper, mashed garlic and parsley into pan drippings and mix well over low heat. If needed, add water to make 1 cup. Cut chicken into strips and lay on cooked pasta or rice and pour over sauce.

Serving Suggestion: Also good with baked potato and a green vegetable such as steamed broccoli, beans or peas.

BARBEQUED CHICKEN

8	chicken thighs, or breasts, skinned and fat cut off
4	garlic cloves, minced
2 tablespoons	garlic oil
2 cups	barbeque sauce (recipe on page 132)

Heat oil in large frying pan that can be put in oven. Add chicken and saute until browned. Drain off any excess oil. Add garlic and stir a few times until lightly browned. Pour sauce over thighs. Cover and place in a 350 degree oven and bake for 45 minutes. Uncover and bake for 15 minutes more.

Note: You don't have to saute chicken and garlic if you want to save time, but it does add a lot of flavor.

STIR FRY CHICKEN AND VEGETABLES

| 4-6 | boneless, skinless chicken breasts, cut in bite sized pieces |

Mix together and put in plastic bag:

1 cup	flour
½ teaspoon	cayenne
½ teaspoon	paprika
1 teaspoon	salt

Shake pieces of chicken in bag a little at a time, dump into large wire strainer and shake over sink or bowl until all excess flour is gone.

In large frying pan or wok add:

1 tablespoon	olive oil
1 tablespoon	butter
1 tablespoon	garlic, minced
2 tablespoons	fresh basil, chopped (or 1 tablespoon dried)

Heat oil and butter until hot and add garlic and basil. Stir until well mixed and add chicken pieces. Brown chicken on both sides. Drain off any oil that remains.

1	red pepper, diced
1 cup	celery, diced
1 cup	carrots, diced
½ cup	chopped dried apricots (optional. Can also used fresh or jarred apricots but add last 5 minutes of cooking)

Add vegetables to chicken and stir until well mixed

Sauce:

1/4 cup	red raspberry balsamic vinegar (Wild Thymes)
1 ½ cup	apricot juice
1/4 teaspoon	cardamom
1/4 teaspoon	cinnamon
1 teaspoon	salt
1 tablespoon	brown sugar

Combine sauce ingredients in a bowl and whisk until smooth. Add to chicken and vegetables and stir. Bring to a boil. Simmer on low boil for 10-15 minutes or until sauce is thickened.

Serving Suggestion: Serve over brown rice or wild rice

ROASTED WHOLE CHICKEN WITH CARROT & ZUCCHINI STUFFING

4-5 pound	whole chicken (clean out, wash and dry inside)
4 tablespoons	butter
4 tablespoons	dried onion flakes
1 teaspoon	garlic, minced
2 teaspoons	fresh tarragon (or 1 teaspoon dried)
2 teaspoon	poultry seasoning
1 teaspoon	salt
½ teaspoon	pepper
2 cups	bread crumbs (homemade bread in Bread section of book or use "good" bread)
2 cups	chopped carrots
2 cups	chopped zucchini
1 tablespoon	butter
	salt and pepper
4 cloves	garlic, peeled and left whole

Melt butter in frying pan and add onion, garlic, tarragon, poultry seasoning, salt and pepper. Saute for a minute and add bread crumbs and mix well. Add carrots and zucchini. Cool a bit and stuff chicken. Pull as much skin over stuffing as you can and toothpick. Rub with a tablespoon of butter, salt and pepper. Put 4 or more cloves of peeled garlic under skin. Cover any exposed stuffing with foil. Place in a roasting pan and bake in a 350 degree oven, covered, for 2- 2 ½ hours. The last 15 minutes uncover to brown. Don't forget the garlic under the skin. Remove and serve with meal, tastes great!

Note: **NEVER** stuff turkey or chicken ahead of time. Do it right before you put in oven, however, you can make the stuffing ahead and store in refrigerator (not too far ahead though, a couple of hours is alright)

ROAST CHICKEN WITH APPLE STUFFING

5 pound	whole natural chicken, clean out inside, wash and dry (or 2 game hens)
2 tablespoons	butter
1 cup	celery, chopped
1 cup	apples, chopped
1 cup	carrots, chopped
1 teaspoon	cardamom
1 teaspoon	salt
2 cups	dried bread crumbs (homemade Wheat or Honey Oatmeal, recipes in Bread section of book or "good" bread)
2 tablespoons	apple juice

Melt butter in large frying pan. Add celery, apples, carrots, cardamom, and salt. Stir until well blended and stir in bread crumbs. Mix in apple juice. Cool a little and stuff in chicken. Place chicken in uncovered roasting pan and bake in a 350 degree oven for 2 hours or until well browned and meat thermometer inserted reads 180. After an hour of roasting, brush on the following glaze:

1 cup	apple juice
1/4 cup	brown sugar

Combine in small saucepan and bring to a boil. Simmer on low boil until mixture is thick and syrupy.

CHICKEN & DUMPLINS FOR TIMMY

1 large	natural whole chicken (wash and clean out inside)
1/4 cup	dried onion flakes
8	whole, peeled garlic cloves
1/4 teaspoon	crushed bay leaves
1 tablespoon	salt
1 teaspoon	pepper
1/8 teaspoon	cayenne
1/4 teaspoon	thyme
6 tablespoons	flour
3/4 cup	milk
1 ½ cups	chopped celery
1 ½ cups	chopped carrots

Place chicken in a large pot. Cover chicken with water. Bring to a boil, cover and simmer for 1 to 1½ hours or until done. Turn over once or twice. Take out chicken and place on cookie sheet or large platter and let cool until you can handle. Place broth in refrigerator while you are getting chicken ready. Pull chicken apart and separate good chicken and throw away the bones and skin, etc. Take broth out of the refrigerator and skim the fat off the top (or use fat separator).Strain broth and measure out 6 cups (freeze the rest of the broth for later use). Put broth back in pot and add onion, garlic, bay leaves, salt, pepper, cayenne and thyme. Mix flour and milk together until smooth. Add to broth in pot and bring to a boil stirring until smooth and thickened. Reduce heat to medium. Add chicken, celery and carrots.

Dumpling Dough: (makes 8-10 dumplings, double as needed)

1	egg
1/3 cup	milk
1 tablespoon	canola or olive oil
3/4 cup	flour
1 tablespoon	fresh or dried parsley
1 teaspoon	baking powder
½ teaspoon	salt
dash	nutmeg

Beat the egg, milk and oil together. Add flour, parsley, baking powder, salt and nutmeg. Drop heaping tablespoons of dumpling dough onto broth. Cover and simmer, without lifting lid, for 15 minutes.

TANGY CHICKEN THIGHS

1 cup	rice vinegar
½ cup	balsamic vinegar (Wild Thymes Red Raspberry)
½ tablespoon	garlic, minced
½ tablespoon	fresh rosemary, finely chopped
8	chicken thighs, skinned, fat cut off, bone removed
1 tablespoon	canola or olive oil

Combine vinegars and garlic and bring to a boil. Continue to cook on low boil until thick and syrupy (takes about 15-20 minutes or so). Stir in rosemary. While sauce is cooking, cook chicken.
Heat oil in a large, heavy oven proof skillet. When oil is hot, add chicken thighs (without the bone, you will need to fold them in half to cook). Season with salt and pepper. Cook on both sides until brown, about 5 minutes. Remove chicken to a platter and drain off any excess fat. Put chicken back in pan. Heat oven to 450 degrees. Transfer pan to oven and roast for 15-20 minutes or until chicken is done. Remove chicken from oven and brush on vinegar mixture. Place under broiler until glaze is bubbly, 1-3 minutes.

FRIED CHICKEN

The best fried chicken I ever had was at my Aunt Pat's in Arkansas. I watched her technique, added some seasonings to the flour, and it is one of my families favorite dinners. I don't make it very often, because of the fat content, but once in a while is okay. The trick to making it a little less "bad" is to take off skin and excess fat and make sure the oil is very hot so it won't be greasy

8	boneless, skinless chicken breasts
10	thighs, skin and excess fat removed (can also remove bones)
3 cups	unbleached all purpose flour
4 teaspoons	garlic powder
2 teaspoons	onion powder
1/4 teaspoon	paprika
5 teaspoons	salt
1/4 teaspoon	poultry seasoning
2 teaspoons	pepper, freshly ground

Place chicken in a deep bowl or pan and cover with milk. Refrigerate at least 2 hours. In a plastic bag mix the flour, garlic powder, onion powder, paprika, salt, poultry seasoning and pepper. Shake ingredients to mix well. Remove one piece of chicken at a time from the milk and place in bag and shake until well coated. Dip the piece into the milk again and shake again. Shake off excess. Place each piece on a cookie sheet lined with wax paper. Let dry for 15 minutes. Heat about a 1/4"-1/2" of canola or olive oil in a very large, deep frying pan. You will need two frying pans with this much chicken or do in batches. Make sure oil is very hot, 365 degrees using a candy thermometer, or when oil sizzles. Add chicken, very carefully, to hot oil. Don't crowd pan too much. Turn down heat but maintain a steady low boil. Lightly brown chicken on both sides. Cover and simmer, turning only once, for approximately 10-15 minutes on each side. Uncover pan and continue to fry, approximately five minutes or until juices from chicken run clear. Place on paper towel lined cookie sheet.

Gravy:

After removing chicken, pour off all of the oil, leaving the browned bits and a 1/4 cup of the oil. Stir flour into remaining oil until you have a smooth paste. Gradually add milk or water, or half of each stirring constantly, until you have the consistency you want. Add salt and pepper to taste.

Serving Suggestion: mashed potatoes are a must with fried chicken and gravy! Corn goes great with it also.

MOM'S ONE PAN CHICKEN DISH

My Mom made this for me when I went to see her recently. I changed it a little making it "trigger free". It's quick and easy and very tasty

½ cup	flour
1/4 teaspoon	paprika
1/4 teaspoon	salt, coarse
1/4 teaspoon	pepper, freshly ground
3 large	chicken breasts
	thyme
1 tablespoon	canola or olive oil
1 tablespoon	butter
1 teaspoon	garlic, minced
2 cups	chicken stock (recipe on page 33)
½ teaspoon	salt
2 large	sweet potatoes or yams, peeled and cut into chunks
3 cups	fresh green beans, de-stringed and broken into bite sized pieces

Mix flour, paprika, salt, pepper on a large plate. Roll chicken breasts in flour mixture to cover both sides. Shake off excess flour. Sprinkle a little thyme on both sides of breasts. Heat butter and oil in a large frying pan. Brown chicken breasts quickly on both sides. Take out chicken and cut into strips. Add garlic to pan and stir a few times until light brown. Pour stock into pan stirring up pan drippings, add salt. Put chicken back into pan. Place sweet potatoes in pan with chicken. Cover and simmer for approximately 30 minutes. Add green beans, cover and simmer for another 10 minutes or until tender.

MOM'S ARROZ CON POLLO (chicken with rice)

14 ounce can	diced tomatoes
1	red pepper (roasted or not)and diced
1/4 cup	onion flakes
2 teaspoons	garlic, minced
½ to 1 teaspoon	salt
1 teaspoon	chili powder
4	boneless, skinless chicken breasts, sprinkle both sides with freshly ground pepper and paprika
½ pound	sausage, optional (recipe on page 61, Hans or Golden Farms) formed into balls
1 cup	peas, frozen
1 cup	brown rice or wild rice, cooked according to package directions

Put tomatoes, red pepper, onion, garlic, salt, and chili in Dutch oven and mix well. Place seasoned chicken and sausage into cooker and cover with sauce. Cover and cook in a 350 degree oven for 1 to 1 ½ hours. The last half hour, add the peas. Serve with rice.

Note: My Mom makes this in a slow cooker (4-6 hours) and adds the rice the last 1-2 hours and the peas the last half hour

CHICKEN CHILI WITH CORN MEAL DUMPLINGS

2	large chicken breasts, diced
1 tablespoon	oil
1 tablespoon	garlic, minced
½ cup	dried onion flakes
1 1/4 teaspoons	cumin
1/8 teaspoon	cayenne
1 teaspoon	chili
3 teaspoons	salt
28 ounces	tomatoes (Eden Organic Diced Tomatoes)
4 cups	water
2	stalks of celery, diced
1/8 cup	cilantro, fresh, chopped
½ cup	leeks, chopped (remove root end and tough green leaves from the top and one or two layers of the rest leaving only the tender part of the leek)
½ cup-1 cup	green chilies, de-seeded, roasted, peeled and diced
1 cup	corn, fresh cut off cob or frozen sweet white corn

In large dutch oven, heat oil. Brown diced chicken in oil. Add garlic, onion, cumin, chili, and salt. Stir until oil is gone. Add tomatoes and water. Add celery, cilantro, leeks, and chilies. Simmer for approximately 30 minutes. Mix dumplings (recipe below) and form into 8 balls. Add corn to soup and stir. Carefully place balls, equal distance apart, on hot stew. Cover pot and simmer on low boil for 20 minutes, don't lift lid. Ladle stew into bowls and sprinkle grated cheese on each portion, if desired.

Dumplings:

1/4 cup	milk
1	egg
1 cup	yellow cornmeal
½ teaspoon	salt
½ teaspoon	baking powder

Beat milk and egg together. Sift cornmeal, salt and baking powder together. Add to milk and egg mixture.

MOTHER'S DAY PEACH CHICKEN

I wanted to make something special for my Mom for Mother's Day, so I came up with this recipe and she loved it!

2 cups	peach juice
2 tablespoons	brown sugar
½ teaspoon	salt
1/4 teaspoon	paprika
½ cup	water
2 tablespoons	flour

Mix peach juice, brown sugar, salt, and paprika. Mix water and flour until smooth. Add to juice mixture. Stir constantly over medium heat until boiling. Continue cooking (low boil) for about 20 minutes until thickened. Prepare chicken while sauce is simmering.

4-6	chicken breasts (boneless, skinless) cut in bite sized pieces (3 cups)
½ cup	unbleached all purpose flour
½ teaspoon	paprika
1/4 teaspoon	cayenne pepper
1 teaspoon	salt
1/4 cup	canola or olive oil
1 tablespoon	butter
1 cup	cut up carrots, peeled and sliced (bite sized pieces)
1 cup	celery, peeled and sliced
1 cup	peaches, fresh, peeled and cut in bite sized pieces (or Heritage Foods, or Del Monte canned peaches)

Mix flour, paprika, cayenne and salt and put in plastic bag. Shake chicken pieces until well coated. Place a few pieces at a time into large wire strainer and shake off excess flour over bowl (re-use flour if needed). Heat oil and butter in large frying pan. When very hot, add chicken pieces and saute until brown on both sides. Take out chicken and drain off any leftover oil. Add sauce to pan and stir up browned bits. Put chicken back in pan. Add carrots and celery. Simmer over medium heat until carrots and celery are done but still crunchy, about 7-10 minutes. Add peaches and cook for another minute.

Serving Suggestion: Great with wild rice and Cucumber Salad (recipe on page 110)

BEEF DISHES

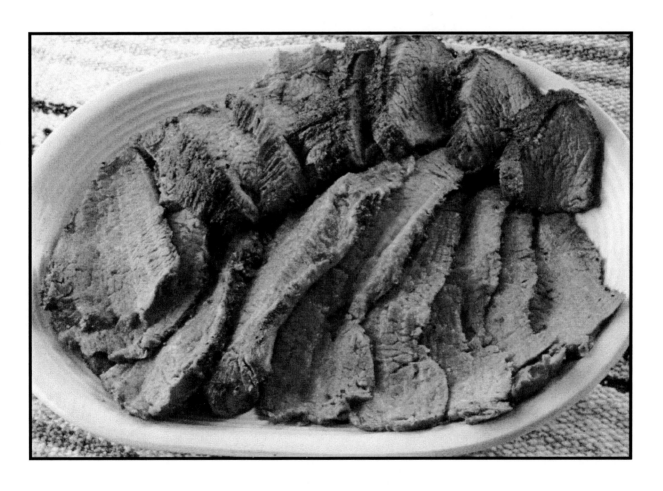

Grilled Tri Tip, page 51

BEEF RUB

This rub is used in several recipes. This combination of spices is great on any grilled beef. Combine spices and put in a jar with a shaker top, sprinkle or rub on both sides of beef before cooking

2 teaspoons	salt
½ teaspoon	paprika
½ teaspoon	cayenne
1 teaspoon	garlic powder
1 teaspoon	onion powder
½ teaspoon	white pepper
1/4 teaspoon	dry mustard
1 teaspoon	chili powder

BEEF STOCK

6 pounds	beef soup bones (or leftover bones from steak, etc.)
½ cup	dried onion flakes
2	carrots, scrubbed and cut up
2 stalks	celery with leaves, cut up
1 large	tomato, cut up
8 whole	peppercorns
4 sprigs	parsley
1	bay leaf
1 clove	garlic, peeled and halved
1 tablespoon	salt, coarse
12 cups	cold water

In a large stock pot or Dutch oven, place the bones, onion, carrots, celery, tomato, peppercorns, parsley, bay leaf, garlic, salt. Add the water and bring to boiling. Reduce heat, cover and simmer for 4 to 5 hours.

Lift out bones with a slotted spoon. Strain the stock through a strainer lined with cheesecloth. Discard the vegetables and seasonings. Skim off the fat with a metal spoon or chill the stock and lift off the solidified fat. Makes about 10 cups of stock.

Note: If you want a richer stock, spread the bones, onions and carrots in a large, shallow roasting pan so that the bones will brown evenly. Bake in a 450 degree oven for 30 minutes, turning the bones occasionally with tongs. Drain off any fat and add all ingredients to pot and cook according to directions above.

Note: If you want to clarify stock, directions are on page 22

DRIED TOMATO MEAT LOAF & RED POTATOES

1 tablespoon	canola or olive oil
½ cup	dried onion flakes
2 teaspoons	garlic, minced
2 teaspoons	fresh basil or 1 teaspoon dried
1 teaspoon	fresh oregano or ½ teaspoon dried
1 teaspoon	pepper
1 teaspoon	salt
½ teaspoon	thyme
1 1/4 cup	dried tomatoes (no sulfur dioxide: Melissa's, Trader Joe's or make your own (recipe on page 22 in Kitchen Techniques section of book)
2 pounds	ground sirloin
1 beaten	egg
20 small	red potatoes, sliced once or twice

Heat oil in small frying pan and add onion, garlic, basil, oregano, pepper, salt and thyme. Stir over low heat until onion is lightly browned and seasonings are well mixed. Set aside. Place tomatoes in small bowl and add 1 cup of boiling water (or a little more if needed to cover tomatoes). Let sit for at least 15 minutes. Pour tomatoes through a strainer into another bowl. Reserve juice. Finely dice tomatoes.

Mix meat with egg, sauteed seasonings, and 1 cup of the tomatoes. Reserve 1/4 cup for the sauce. Mix meat mixture with hands to blend in seasonings well, and form into loaf. Place in a 9" x 13" baking pan. Place sliced red potatoes around loaf. Add ½ cup water to pan. Bake in a 375 degree oven for 1 to 1 hour and 15 minutes. Occasionally turn potatoes for even browning and add more water if needed. Take meatloaf and potatoes out of pan and put on platter. Cover with foil to keep warm.

Sauce:

Pour reserved liquid from tomatoes into pan used to bake meatloaf. Stir in 2 tablespoons of flour until smooth. Add 1 teaspoon salt and 1/4 teaspoon pepper. Gradually add ½ cup of milk stirring constantly over medium low heat until smooth and thickened (add more milk or water if you like thinner). Add finely diced reserved 1/4 cup of dried tomatoes. Serve over meatloaf or on the side.

SWEET & SOUR MEATBALLS

2 pounds	ground sirloin (or very lean ground beef) or: 1 pound ground sirloin and 1 pound ground pork
1	egg, beaten
½ cup	dried onion flakes
1/4 teaspoon	paprika
1/8 teaspoon	cayenne
½ teaspoon	pepper, freshly ground
1 teaspoon	salt
½ teaspoon	ginger
1 or 2	red peppers, de-seeded, roasted, and diced (roasting optional)
1 large	apple, peeled, cored and diced

Mix together with your hands, beef, egg, onion, paprika, cayenne, pepper, salt and ginger until well blended. To make meatballs of equal size, pat meat mixture into a 1" thick rectangle. Cut the rectangle into equal squares, the size you want (small bite size, I think, are best). Gently roll in your hand, each square, into a smooth ball without cracks. Lightly spray large frying pan with a little oil and place meatballs in pan. Cover and simmer on medium low heat until brown, turn to brown other side. Place meatballs on a plate, cover to keep warm. Drain off any excess oil in pan.

Sauce:

½ cup	brown sugar
1 cup	apple juice
1½ cups	brown rice vinegar or rice vinegar or a combination of both
1/4 teaspoon	salt
½ teaspoon	ginger
2 tablespoons	water
2 tablespoons	flour

Blend together in saucepan: brown sugar, juice, vinegar, salt, and ginger. Mix the water and flour together in a small cup and mix until smooth. Add to mixture in saucepan. Bring to a boil, stirring constantly. Lower heat and cook until thickened. Pour sauce into the frying pan that you cooked the meatballs in. Stir up brown bits in pan. Put meatballs back in pan, add diced red pepper and apple. Bring to a boil, turn down heat, gently stir and simmer just until meatballs are coated with sauce and heated through. Serve over rice.

CABBAGE AND BEEF CASSEROLE

1 pound	ground sirloin or lean ground beef or ground turkey
1 tablespoon	garlic, minced
1 tablespoon	dried oregano or basil (or 2 tablespoons fresh)
1/4 cup	dried onion flakes
1 teaspoon	onion powder
1 tablespoon	mustard (recipe on page 129 or Rothschild)
1/4 teaspoon	cayenne
½ teaspoon	paprika
½ teaspoon	salt
½ teaspoon	pepper
28 ounces	tomatoes (Eden Organic crushed or diced) if whole, blend
1	cabbage
2 cups	farmer cheese, grated (may-bud)

Saute meat until brown and drain off extra liquid. Add garlic, oregano or basil, onion flakes, onion powder, mustard, cayenne, paprika, salt and pepper. Add tomatoes and simmer for 30-40 minutes until very thick (the moisture of the cabbage adds a lot of liquid).

Discard outer leaves of cabbage, tear off inside leaves and cut into bite size pieces. Cover the bottom of an 8" x 11" lightly oiled baking pan with half cabbage. Spoon half of sauce over cabbage, then sprinkle half of the cheese over the sauce. Repeat layers and end with cheese. Bake in a 350 degree oven for 40 minutes.

MEATBALLS AND SAUCE

2 pounds	ground sirloin, very lean ground beef, or natural pork sausage (sausage recipe on page 61, or Hans or Golden Farms) or a combination of beef and pork
1	red pepper, finely diced
½ cup	dried onion flakes
1/4 teaspoon	paprika
1/8 teaspoon	cayenne
½ teaspoon	white pepper
1 teaspoon	salt
1 teaspoon	dried oregano

Mix together with hands until well blended. Make into medium size balls rolling in your hands to make smooth (no cracks). Spray large frying pan with a little oil and place meatballs close together in pan. Cover and simmer on medium low heat until brown. Turn to brown on the other side. While meatballs are cooking, make sauce.

Sauce:

5 cups	fresh tomatoes, pulse in blender so you have some chunks
12 ounces	tomato paste (optional, if you like a thicker sauce)
2 tablespoons	fresh basil (or 1 tablespoon dried)
4 tablespoons	fresh oregano (or 2 tablespoon dried)
4	garlic cloves, minced
½ teaspoon	salt
1 cup	water

Bring ingredients to a boil stirring to blend. Lower heat, cover and simmer for 30 minutes or until thickened. Add sauce to meatballs. Serve over pasta.

50

GRILLED TRI TIP

I had never heard of tri tip until my son-in-law, Brian, made it for us. It was so delicious that it has become a family favorite. Another great way to cook this meat is to marinate it (recipe at the bottom of the page)

Tri tip sprinkled or rubbed with Beef Rub (recipe on page 47)

Grill and use meat thermometer to determine when it is done to your liking. Thinly slice, at an angle, across the grain.

Serving Suggestion: Great with Mashed Potatoes (recipe on page 95) and corn on the cob or Grilled Vegetables (recipe on page 101

MARINATED AND GRILLED LONDON BROIL

2 pound   London broil, tri tip or flank steak

Marinade:

1/4 cup	roasted red pepper oil (Consorzio) olive or canola oil
1/4 cup	vinegar (Wild Thymes Cranberry Ginger Balsamic Vinegar)
1/4 cup	cranberry juice
1 tablespoon	brown sugar
1 tablespoon	grated fresh ginger (I keep it in the freezer, it peels and grates easier and stays fresh a long time. Cut off a piece, peel and grate as needed.

Mix together marinade in a pan about the size of the meat. Place meat in pan and pour marinade on top. Cover and put in refrigerator. Turn every few hours and coat well. Best if marinated over night but a few hours is fine. Throw away marinade and grill to your liking using a meat thermometer. Cool a little and thinly slice, at an angle, across the grain.

STUFFED ROUND STEAK

| large | round steak, thinly cut (or carefully pound until thin) |

Marinade:

12 ounces	apple juice
1/8 cup	balsamic vinegar
1 tablespoon	brown sugar
1 teaspoon	dry mustard
1 teaspoon	olive or canola oil

Mix the juice, vinegar, brown sugar, dry mustard and oil together in a shallow pan. Place round steak in pan, the liquid should cover steak. Cover tightly and marinate in the refrigerator overnight.

Stuffing:

2 tablespoons	butter
1 teaspoon	canola or olive oil
1 teaspoon	garlic
2 tablespoons	dried onion flakes
1 tablespoon	basil, finely chopped fresh (or ½ tablespoon dried)
1/4 teaspoon	paprika
1/4 teaspoon	salt
1/4 teaspoon	pepper
1 cup	jicama, finely chopped
1 cup	celery, finely chopped

Melt butter in small frying pan and add oil. Add garlic, onion, basil, paprika, salt and pepper and stir a few times. Add jicama and celery and stir until well blended. Put into bowl to cool.

Lay the marinated steak flat on a clean work surface, and spoon stuffing down the middle of the steak, not too close to edges. Discard marinade. Roll steak tightly and tie with cotton string (or toothpicks) to hold. Tuck in ends and toothpick. Place in baking pan, just big enough for roll. Add water to cover the bottom of the pan. Cover and bake for approximately 1 ½ hours. Check every 30 minutes to make sure there is enough liquid, add water if necessary. Place roll on plate. Strain the pan drippings into a small sauce pan (you should have a cup of liquid, add water to make a cup, if needed). In a small cup, stir 1 tablespoon of flour into 2 tablespoons of water and stir until smooth. Add to pan of drippings. Stir over medium heat until smooth and thickened. Add salt and pepper to taste (about 1/4 teaspoon of each). Slice roll into servings and drizzle sauce over or serve on the side.

BRAISED ROUND STEAK AND POTATOES

Cut off any fat on steak and cut in serving size portions. Rub flour on both sides of meat. Heat olive or canola oil, only enough to cover the bottom of a large oven proof skillet. When oil is hot, saute steak on medium high heat until browned, turn over and brown other side. Sprinkle with salt and freshly ground pepper. Remove from pan after browning both sides. Add two cups of water to pan and stir up pan drippings. Put the round steak back in pan.

Scrub and cut up potatoes (small red or new potatoes or russet cut in bit sized pieces) and place on top of steak. Sprinkle potatoes with salt and pepper. Cover pan and place in a 350 degree oven for approximately 1- 1 ½ hours until meat is tender and potatoes are done. Check every 20 minutes or so to make sure there is still plenty of liquid in pan. Add water if needed. Remove steak and potatoes to a platter, stir up pan drippings and pour on top.

CHILE STUFFED FLANK STEAK

	flank steak at least 3/4" thick
4 or 5	green chiles (Anaheim) cut off top, carefully remove seeds, leave whole, roast (broil approximately 6 minutes each side until black, put in plastic or paper bag for 10 minutes and peel)
5 tablespoons	farmer cheese
1 teaspoon	salt and pepper
2 teaspoons	olive oil

To form a pocket in the steak, lay the steak flat on cutting board. Using a very sharp knife, stick knife in the side of steak, about 1" from the end. Slowly cut through the middle working very carefully so you won't cut through the back. Cut 1" from the other end.

Stuff the chilies with a tablespoon of cheese. Place chiles in pocket of steak and skewer the open end. Rub a teaspoon of oil and salt and pepper on each side of steak. Grill steak until done to your liking. Let rest for 5 minutes. Slice across grain with a very sharp knife.

Serving Suggestion: Great with Spanish rice (make your favorite rice and add salsa)

SLOW SIMMERED FLANK STEAK
This recipe can also be made in a slow cooker. Quick and easy and tastes great.

2 pound	flank steak
1 tablespoon	olive or canola oil
1/3 cup	dried onion flakes
½ tablespoon	fresh garlic minced
1 cup	water
2 tablespoons	rice vinegar
1 teaspoon	chili powder
½ teaspoon	sugar
1 teaspoon	salt
½ teaspoon	pepper
½ cup	green chiles, de-seeded, roasted, peeled and chopped

Heat oil in large oven proof skillet and brown steak on both sides. Place on plate. In the same skillet stir onion and garlic a few times to lightly brown. Add water stirring to loosen browned bits from pan. Add remaining ingredients, except green chiles, and stir until well blended. Put steak back in pan, or in slow cooker. Pour sauce ingredients on top of steak leaving most of the onions and garlic on top of steak. Put diced chiles on top of steak. Cook on low for 5-6 hours in slow cooker or in covered oven proof skillet in a 300 degree oven for approximately 3-4 hours or until tender. Check every hour or so and add more water if needed. Thinly slice meat, at an angle, across the grain and serve with pan juices.

Serving Suggestion: Serve with noodles, rice, mashed potatoes or bread and a steamed vegetable.

BEEF STEW

2 pounds	lean stew meat
1/4 cup	dried onion flakes
1/4 cup	minced parsley
½ teaspoon	oregano
1 teaspoon	margoram
1 teaspoon	salt
2 cups	water
28 ounces	crushed or diced tomatoes (Eden Organics)

cut up potatoes (I like to use small red potatoes or new potatoes) and carrots (how ever many you need for your family) Add any other vegetables you like: corn, cabbage, etc.

Cut stew meat into bite size pieces, place in plastic bag with flour and shake to coat pieces, place meat into large strainer over sink and shake off excess flour. Heat oil in a large stew pot (just enough oil to cover bottom of pot). Stir and brown meat. Add 2 cups of water and stir up pan drippings. Add tomatoes and stir. Simmer on low (just bubbling a little) for 1 hour Add potatoes and carrots and cook until done (about another hour, test after 30 minutes and again at 45 minutes)

SWISS STEAK

This is a very simple and tasty recipe. Round steak is a very lean cut of meat and usually inexpensive. This would also be a good recipe for the crock pot, just make sure you add enough liquid

1 tablespoon	olive oil
1/4 cup	dried onion flakes
2 teaspoons	garlic, minced
1	lean round steak (cut off all fat and slice in serving size portions)
	salt and pepper to taste
14 ounces	diced tomatoes (Eden Organic or fresh)
½ cup	water, more as needed

Heat oil in medium oven proof frying pan or dutch oven. When oil is hot, saute meat until browned on both sides. Remove meat to a plate. Add onion, and garlic to pan and saute over low heat until slightly browned. Add tomatoes to pan and stir with garlic and onion. Put back meat and sprinkle with salt and pepper. Place covered pan in a 350 degree oven for approximately 1 ½ hours. Add sliced potatoes or small red or new potatoes and cook for another 45 minutes or until meat and potatoes are tender. Check every 20 minutes and add water as needed.

CROSS RIB ROAST, POTATOES, CARROTS AND GRAVY

This is a great company dish. Everyone loves it and it is so simple and delicious.

4 pound	cross rib roast (3/4 pound per person)
3-4 tablespoons	canola or olive oil (enough to just cover the bottom of the pan)
½ cup	dried onion flakes
1 tablespoon	garlic, minced
	coarse salt & freshly ground pepper
4	potatoes, peeled and quartered
6 large	carrots, peeled or scrubbed and cut in bite size pieces

Heat oil, medium low heat, in Dutch oven. Add roast and brown on both sides. Add garlic and onions and stir a few times to brown lightly. Salt and pepper roast. Add 2 cups of water and place, covered, in a 350 degree oven (takes approximately 4 hours) After an hour, turn roast and add water if needed. Set timer for 1 hour and turn again and add water if necessary. Repeat. Add peeled potatoes cut in quarters and cut up carrots, place around roast. Cook for another hour or until roast is very tender and vegetables are done. Take out meat and vegetables (keep warm covered with foil). Stir flour into pan drippings to make a thick paste (no heat). Add water a little at a time and stir constantly over medium heat. Keep adding water until gravy is the thickness that you like and is very well blended and bubbling. Add 1 teaspoon of salt or to taste.

Serving Suggestion: My family likes this roast with Mashed Potatoes (recipe on page 95) and corn instead of the roasted potatoes and carrots.

BEEF STROGANOFF

1 large	round steak or other lean beef
1 teaspoon	oil
1 teaspoon	butter
3/4 teaspoon	salt, coarse
1/4 teaspoon	pepper, freshly ground
2 tablespoons	dried onion
2 cups	water
2 teaspoons	mustard (recipe on page 129 or Rothschild)
1/4 cup	water
1 tablespoon	flour
1/8 teaspoon	paprika
8 ounces	sour cream, Daisy
8 ounces	noodles, cooked according to package directions

Cut all the fat off of the meat and slice in thin bite sized strips. Heat oil and butter and saute meat on both sides until browned and almost all the liquid is gone. Add the salt, pepper and onion. Stir a few times. Mix together 1 cup of water and the mustard. Add to the pan. Stir, cover and simmer for approximately 1 hour and 15 minutes. Check after 30 minutes and if needed, add another cup of water. Mix 1/4 cup water, flour and paprika together. When meat is tender, add the water mixture to the pan and stir until well mixed and thickened. Add more water if needed to make the right consistency. Stir in the sour cream just until well blended and hot, don't boil. Serve immediately over cooked noddles.

PORK DISHES

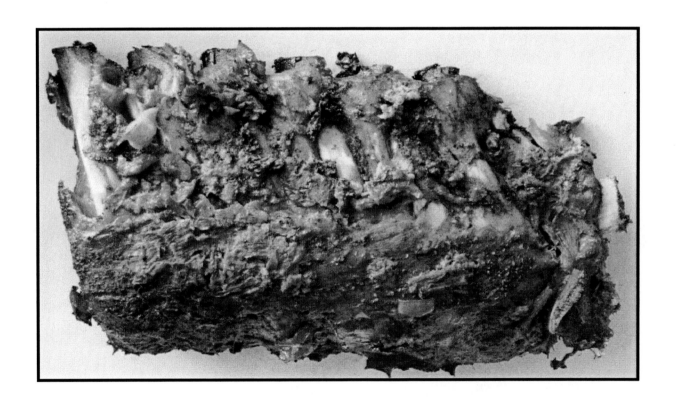

Slow Cooked and Marinated Baby Back Ribs, page 60

PORK RUB

This rub is used in several recipes. Mix spices together, put in jar with shaker top and sprinkle or rub on pork before cooking

2 teaspoons	salt
½ teaspoon	paprika
1/8 teaspoon	cayenne
1 teaspoon	parsley
1/4 teaspoon	white pepper

SHREDDED PORK OR BEEF BARBEQUE

6-7 pounds	center cut pork loin, pork sirloin, or fresh pork shoulder roast
	fat removed
	barbeque sauce (recipe on page 132)

Melt oil in the bottom of a very large oven proof frying pan and add trimmed pork. Sprinkle with salt and pepper. Brown on high heat until browned on both sides. Drain off all oil and add a cup or two of water. You can simmer it on top of the stove or in a 350 degree oven. You will need to add water every 20 minutes or so. Check often so it won't boil dry. It will take about 3 to 4 hours to become very tender. Take out and let cool until you can handle and shred. Lay in pan. Pour sauce over (to taste), cover and cook in a 350 degree oven for about 45 minutes to an hour.

BARBEQUE RIBS

pork loin country style ribs or beef ribs
barbeque sauce (recipe on page 132)

Place ribs in large pot and cover with water. Bring to a boil. Turn down heat so they are gently simmering. Simmer for 1 hour. Place ribs in heavy roasting pan and cover with sauce. Bake for approximately 1 hour or until tender. Or, cover with sauce, place on foil and grill.

Baby Back Ribs
Cut racks into 3 and 4 rib sections. Coat the bottom of a roasting pan with enough barbeque sauce to cover. Add ribs to pan and coat with sauce. Bake in a 325 degree oven until ribs are cooked through, about an hour. Start a charcoal or gas grill (discard sauce remaining in pan). Grill ribs turning and basting frequently with more sauce until well browned and heated through, 10-15 minutes. Heat extra sauce on stove to serve with ribs.

Note:	My son-in-law, Brian, adds coconut to his barbeque sauce and it really adds a great flavor.

SPICED APPLESAUCE PORK ROAST

4-6 pound	boneless pork loin roast
2 large	garlic cloves, skinned, cut in thin lengthwise strips
1 tablespoon	mustard (recipe on page 129 or Rothschild)
1 cup	applesauce (recipe on page 134 or "good" applesauce)
1/3 cup	brown sugar
2 teaspoons	apple cider vinegar
1/8 teaspoon	ground cloves

Cut off any fat from roast. Cut long slit in top of roast and insert garlic strips. Rub the mustard evenly all over roast. Place in a roasting pan and bake in a 325 degree oven for 30-40 minutes per pound or until meat thermometer tests done. Combine applesauce, brown sugar, vinegar and cloves. Spoon over meat during the last half hour of baking.

Serving Suggestion: Great with Sweet Potato Casserole (recipe on page 97)

CRANBERRY PORK ROAST

1 cup	water
½ cup	brown sugar
2 cups	apple juice
12 ounces	whole, fresh cranberries
2 teaspoons	mustard (recipe on page 129 or Rothschild) or dry mustard
1/4 teaspoon	ground cloves
2 pound	boneless pork loin or rib end roast

Bring water, sugar and juice to a boil. Add cranberries and return to boiling. Simmer (low boil) for 10 minutes until tender, whisk to break up cranberries. Add mustard and cloves and continue to cook until thickened. Pour sauce through strainer to remove any cranberry skins.

Place roast in heavy roasting pan and coat roast with about a cup of sauce. Reserve the rest for serving. Pour water in pan just to cover bottom. Place oven rack in upper third of oven. Cover and bake in a 350 degree oven for approximately 2 ½ - 3 hours. Check once or twice during cooking and add water to pan if necessary and baste roast with sauce. Slice and serve with hot sauce.

Note: If you like a lot of sauce, you can double the sauce recipe, baste with half of it and reserve the other half for serving with pork.

APRICOT GLAZED PORK CHOPS AND FRUITED RICE

1 tablespoon	butter
1/4 cup	dried onion flakes
½ cup	uncooked brown rice
1 tablespoon	parsley
½ teaspoon	sage
½ teaspoon	salt
½ cup	dried apricots, diced
1 cup	apricot juice
1 1/3 cup	water
½ cup	apricot preserves (Hero)
1/8 teaspoon	Tabasco pepper sauce (or just a dash if you don't want it too hot)
4	pork chops, center cut boneless

Melt butter over low heat, add onion and saute for a minute. Add rice, parsley, sage, salt and apricots. Saute another minute. Add juice and water. Bring to a boil. Cover and simmer on low heat until rice is tender, about 40-50 minutes. Check every 15 minutes and add water (1/2 cup) if needed. Cook until almost dry. Make sure the rice is tender.

While the rice is simmering, put apricot preserves and pepper sauce in a small sauce pan and stir until hot and well blended. Salt and pepper pork chops and grill until done. You can also do chops in the oven. Line bottom of broiler pan with foil. Spray top of broiler pan with oil and place chops. Bake in a 375 degree oven for 40 minutes. The last 10 minutes spread half of the apricot preserve mixture on top of the chops. Add the other half of the apricot mixture to the rice mixture and stir until well blended.

OVEN BAKED PORK CHOPS

1 tablespoon	olive oil
4-6	center cut pork chops, trim fat off of edges
1 teaspoon	garlic, minced
2 tablespoons	dried onion flakes
4-6	center cut pork chops, trim fat off of edges
14 ounce	diced tomatoes (Eden Organic or fresh)
2 teaspoons	fresh basil, chopped (1 teaspoon dried)
2 teaspoons	fresh oregano (1 teaspoon dried)
½ teaspoon	salt
½ teaspoon	pepper, freshly ground
3-4 cups	small red or new potatoes, scrubbed and cut in half

Heat oil in large oven proof frying pan. Saute pork chops until browned. Take out pork chops and add garlic and onions and stir for a second or two. Add tomatoes, basil, oregano, salt, and pepper. Stir until well mixed and put pork chops back in pan. Spoon some of the sauce on top of the chops. Place potatoes on top of pork chops. Bake in 350 degree oven for approximately 1-1 ½ hours until chops and potatoes are tender . Check every 30 minutes to make sure there is enough liquid. Add water if needed.

Serving Suggestion: This dish is also good with a baked potato or baked sweet potato or yam. Or, slice yams or sweet potatoes, place in heavy duty foil, put a little butter on top and wrap tightly. Place on rack beside the chops and they will be done at the same time.

GRILLED PORK, SWEET POTATOES AND APPLES

| 2 pound | pork loin sprinkled with Pork Rub (recipe on page 56) |

Place pork on two layers of heavy duty foil, cover with two more pieces the same size and tightly roll and seal edges.

3	long, narrow sweet potatoes, peeled and sliced
4 tablespoons	melted butter
1 teaspoon	salt

Mix together potatoes, butter and salt. Place on 2 layers of heavy duty foil. Cover with two more pieces of foil the same size and tightly roll and seal edges.

6	Granny Smith apples, cored, peeled and sliced
1 teaspoon	cinnamon
½ cup	sugar

Mix together apples, cinnamon and sugar. Place on 2 layers of heavy duty foil. Cover with two more pieces of foil the same size and tightly roll and seal edges.

Place pork and sweet potato packages on grill and cook on low heat, top shelf, closed grill. After 20 minutes place apple package on grill and turn sweet potato package over. Cook another 20 minutes or until pork is done (no pink) and potatoes are tender. Of course, all grills cook differently so you need to check often and make a note for next time.

STOVE TOP ROASTED PORK WITH LEEKS

3 large	leeks, remove root end, and tough green leaves from the top, and one or two layers of the rest leaving only the tender part of the leek. Rinse, drain well and slice
½ tablespoon	butter
1/4 teaspoon	salt
1/4 teaspoon	pepper
½ tablespoon	butter
1 teaspoon	canola oil
2 pound	boneless pork loin, fat trimmed off
½ cup	water
1/4 teaspoon	salt
1/4 teaspoon	pepper

Place the leeks in a Dutch oven and cover with water. Add the butter, salt and pepper. Cook for 10 minutes or until leeks have wilted. Pour water and leeks into a bowl. Heat butter and oil in the same pan. Add pork and brown on all sides. Take out pork and add ½ cup of the reserved leek water to pan stirring up browned bits. Put pork back in pan and sprinkle with salt and pepper. Add leek mixture. The water should come up about half way on the roast. If needed, add more water. Cover and simmer for about 2-2 1/4 hours or until pork is tender and most of the liquid is gone (you should have about a cup left). Check often during cooking to make sure there is enough liquid. Add water if needed. Slice pork and serve with leek sauce.

PORK CHOPS WITH RASPBERRY/APPLE SAUCE & SWEET POTATOES

1 tablespoon	canola or olive oil
4-6	pork chops, boneless, excess fat removed
1	red pepper, de-seeded and chopped
1	apple, peeled, cored and chopped
1 cup	celery, peeled and chopped
½ teaspoon	cinnamon
½ teaspoon	nutmeg
1 teaspoon	salt
1 tablespoon	brown sugar
1 cup	apple juice
½ cup	raspberries (fresh or frozen)
1 or 2	sweet potatoes or yams, peeled and thickly sliced (same size)

In a large frying pan, heat oil and brown pork chops on both sides. Take out chops. Add red peppers, apples, celery, cinnamon, nutmeg, salt, brown sugar, apple juice and raspberries to pan. Stir up browned bits and put back pork chops. Place potatoes on top of chops. Simmer on low heat for about 30-40 minutes. Check once in a while to make sure there is still enough liquid, add more apples juice if needed. Take off lid and simmer for another 10-15 minutes or until chops are tender and liquid has boiled down. Place pork chops and potatoes on platter and spoon over sauce.

Note: You can bake the potatoes in the oven, if you prefer, in a 400 degree oven for 45 minutes.

SLOW COOKED AND MARINATED BABY BACK RIBS

5 pounds	baby back ribs (2 large racks), cut in half so they will fit in pan side by side
	Spice Hunter Steak, Chop, Grill and Broil Seasoning or Beef Rub, recipe on page 47
5-6 large cloves	garlic, minced
4-6 large	green chilies, de-seeded, roasted, peeled and chopped

Rub seasoning evenly on both sides of ribs, to taste. Rub minced garlic on meat to taste. Line a 10 x 15 roasting pan with heavy duty foil the length and width of the pan leaving enough foil to wrap over the ribs and seal. Place the ribs side by side. Sprinkle the chopped green chilies on top of the ribs. Bring the edges of the foil together and tightly seal. Marinate in the refrigerator for 12-24 hours. Remove the pan from the refrigerator for 30 minutes. Cook in a 300 degree oven for 5-6 hours until very tender.

Note: You can also use boneless pork loin ribs

SAUSAGE

1 ½ pounds	ground pork (or you can use ground turkey)
½ teaspoon	salt
1 teaspoon	garlic powder
1/4 teaspoon	pepper, freshly ground
1 teaspoon	paprika
1/4 teaspoon	sage
1/4 teaspoon	anise seed
½ teaspoon	fennel seed
1/4 teaspoon	cayenne

Mix together in a large bowl: pork, salt, garlic, pepper, paprika, sage, anise, fennel and cayenne. Mix with your hands to work the seasonings into the meat until well blended. Form meat into a log and place into large zipper plastic bag. Refrigerate for 12 hours to let the flavors mix.

Cut meat into patties and saute until browned and thoroughly cooked.

Note: Freeze individual patties and use as needed.

Serving Suggestion: Great with Egg White Omelet (recipe on page 89)

FISH DISHES

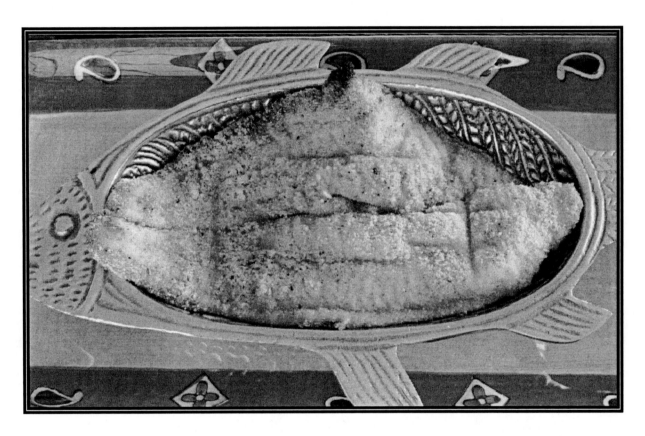

Grilled Catfish Filet, page 63

COOKING TECHNIQUES FOR FISH

Timing is all important when it comes to cooking fish. Perfectly cooked fish is moist and has a delicate flavor, overcooked fish is dry and tasteless. The "10 Minute Rule" is still the best guide to cooking fish by conventional methods. Here's how to use it.

1. Measure the fish at its thickest point. If the fish is stuffed or rolled, measure it after stuffing or rolling, and time it accordingly.
2. Cook fish 10 minutes per inch, turning it halfway through the cooking time. For example, a 1 inch fish steak should be cooked 5 minutes on each side for a total of 10 minutes. Pieces of fish less than ½ inch thick do not have to be turned over.
3. Add 5 minutes to the total cooking time if you are cooking the fish in foil, or if fish is cooked in a sauce.
4. Double the cooking time for frozen fish that has not been defrosted.

Below are some basic cooking techniques for fish:

Baking: Preheat oven to 375 degrees. Bake uncovered, basting if desired.

Oven Broiling: Place fish that is 1 inch thick or less 2 to 4 inches from the heat source; place thicker pieces 5 to 6 inches away. Baste frequently. Cook on one side for half the total cooking time (10 Minute Rule), turn over and continue broiling and basting. Thin filets do not have to be turned over.

Pan Frying or Sauteing: Dip the fish in flour, batter or breading just before frying, if desired. Heat a small amount of oil, or butter or a mixture of both in a pan until very hot, but not smoking (set electric skillet at 350 degrees). Fry for half the total cooking time as determined by the 10 Minute Rule, turn and complete cooking. Fillets less than ½ inch thick do not need to be turned.

. . . .

When choosing fish, make sure it is as fresh as possible. Buy from your butcher and ask to smell it. Shrimp have no smell at all, or very little. No fish should have a strong smell. It's best to buy shrimp uncooked because they are so easily over-cooked and buying in the shell have more flavor. Look at bone line in fish, should be red, not brown. Tuna's flesh should look almost beefy and full, if it is marked "sashimmi quality", meaning it can be eaten raw, it is a good indication of freshness. When buying fresh lobster, ask how long it has been in the tank. Don't buy if very long in tank. Monk fish is great, tastes like lobster!

FISH RUB

This rub is used in several recipes. Combine spices and put in jar with a shaker top, sprinkle on both sides of fish

2 teaspoons	salt
½ teaspoon	cayenne pepper
1 teaspoon	paprika
2 teaspoons	lemon pepper

FISH TACOS

large fresh	fish filet (mild white fish such as: tuna, cod, orange roughy) rubbed with Fish Rub (recipe above) or Spice Hunter Fish Seasoning and grilled
2 cups	cabbage, shredded
1/3 to ½ cup	mayonnaise (recipe on page 129)
1/3 cup	creme fraiche (Vermont Butter and Cream) or sour cream (Daisy)
1 tablespoon	mustard (recipe on page 129 or Rothschild)
2 tablespoons	cilantro, fresh, chopped
1/4 teaspoon	Spice Hunter fish seasoning or Fish Rub (recipe above)
	flour tortillas (recipe on page 72)
	tomatoes, fresh, chopped

Cut the grilled fish into small pieces. Mix the cabbage, mayonnaise, creme fraiche, mustard, cilantro and seasoning. Place the fish slightly to one side of the open tortilla. Fold over and brown on both sides in large frying pan or stove top grill until crispy. Spoon some of the cabbage mixture on top of fish and top with chopped tomatoes.

GRILLED CATFISH FILET

1 large	catfish filet (enough for 2 people)
2 teaspoons	lemongrass ginger oil (Stonewall Kitchen)
½ cup	corn meal
½ teaspoon	salt
½ teaspoon	pepper
1 teaspoon	Fish Rub (recipe above) or Spice Hunter Fish Seasoning

Rub 1 teaspoon oil on each side of fish. Mix together cornmeal, salt, pepper, and seasoning. Rub half on each side of filet .Place filet on foil, or fish basket and grill or rotisserie (using the Cooking Techniques at beginning of chapter) until fish flakes with fork.

Serving Suggestion: Great served with Corn Relish or Cole Slaw (recipes on page 103 and 110) and crusty French Bread (page 120).

GRILLED SALMON & VEGETABLES

I was using heavy duty foil for this recipe and my friend Gail told me about these great foil cooking bags. They are much stronger than foil sheets and do a great job!

1 ½ pound	salmon filet, black & grey skin removed on underside, rubbed with a little lemongrass oil and sprinkled with Fish Rub (recipe on page 63) and 1-2 teaspoons of finely chopped fresh dill
4 cups	small red potatoes, cut in half
1 cup	green beans, cut in bite size pieces
1 cup	small yellow or butternut squash, peeled, de-seeded and cut in bite size pieces
2 tablespoons	butter, melted
1 teaspoon	salt
½ teaspoon	freshly ground pepper
1 tablespoon	fresh dill, chopped

Place salmon in heavy duty foil cooking bag (Reynolds Hot Bags, extra heavy duty large size). Place potatoes, beans and squash in large bowl. Add melted butter, salt, pepper and dill. Mix together and place in bag with salmon. Fold edge of bag over twice and place on preheated grill, top shelf on medium, closed for about 30-40 minutes (depending on your particular grill). With potholders place foil bag on cookie sheet. Carefully slit open and serve immediately.

Serving Suggestion: Great with Fish Dipping Sauces (recipes on page 133). Also good with Cole Slaw (recipe on page 110)

SALMON PASTA

1 pound	salmon filet, gray skin removed on underside, rubbed with Spice Hunter Fish Seasoning or Fish Rub (page 63)
2 tablespoons	butter
1 tablespoon	dried basil or 2 tablespoons fresh
1 teaspoon	fresh lemon balm
1 teaspoon	fresh garlic, minced
½ teaspoon	salt
½ teaspoon	pepper, freshly ground
8 ounce	creme fraiche (Vermont Butter and Cream) or sour cream (Daisy) or use another cup of milk
1 cup	milk
	pasta, cooked according to directions

Melt butter in small saucepan and add basil, lemon balm, garlic, salt and pepper and saute for about a minute. Stir in creme fraiche until well blended. Add milk slowly stirring constantly until thickened. Add bite size pieces of grilled salmon to hot sauce. Serve over cooked pasta

Note: If you are using 2 cups of milk instead of the creme fraiche, thicken with 2 tablespoons of flour (stir in with ingredients in pan before adding milk)

SALMON CAKES

I buy a nice big salmon filet and make the Grilled Salmon (recipe on page 63) and the next night
I make these Salmon Cakes with 2 cups of leftover salmon

2 cups	grilled, flaked salmon
½ cup	corn meal or Old Fashioned Quaker Oats (or ½ of each)
2 tablespoons	milk
2	egg whites, slightly beaten
2 tablespoons	dried onion flakes
2 tablespoons	fresh chopped dill or 1 tablespoon dried dill
1/4 teaspoon	salt

Combine the grilled salmon, corn meal or oats, milk, egg whites, onions, dill and salt. Let stand for 5 minutes, then shape into patties. Spray a large skillet with canola or olive oil and heat. Place patties in hot oil and cook until golden brown on both sides. Makes about 6 medium sized patties.

Serving Suggestion: Serve with one of the Fish Dipping Sauces (page 133) and Red Potatoes & Veggies (recipe on page 96) and Cole Slaw (recipe on page 110).

Note: If you use canned salmon, drain very well and very carefully dump out salmon into the palm of your hand, it should stay together. Then carefully scrape off the gray skin. Open up the salmon and you then can take out the backbone and other bones. Carefully pick through it and only use the desirable pieces.

SALMON CAKES II

2 cups	grilled, flaked salmon
2 large	eggs, beaten
4 tablespoons	mayonnaise (recipe on page 129)
2 tablespoons	mustard (recipe on page 129 or Rothschild)
1/4 teaspoon	cayenne
½ teaspoon	pepper, freshly ground
½ teaspoon	salt
2 tablespoons	dried onion flakes
2 tablespoons	fresh lemon balm, finely chopped, or 1 tablespoon dried (or use cilantro or parsley or a combination of both)
2 cups	"good" bread crumbs (finely processed)

Mix eggs, mayonnaise, mustard, cayenne, pepper, salt. Stir in onions, lemon balm, and bread crumbs. Add grilled, flaked salmon. Let stand for 5 minutes, then shape into patties. Spray a large skillet with canola or olive oil and heat. Place patties in hot oil and cook until golden brown on both sides. Makes about 6 medium sized patties.

Note: You could also use crab in both of these recipes, fresh or canned.

WAYNE'S SPECIAL SALMON

Choose a fresh salmon filet and remove grey skin on underside. Rub filet with a little olive oil. Mix together 1/4 cup to a ½ cup of brown sugar (depending on the size of the filet), a little cayenne, salt and pepper. Rub into salmon on top side. Let sit for 5-10 minutes. Preheat grill for 5 minutes. Place filet on lightly oiled grill guard or foil (coated side up). Grill until salmon flakes.

MARINATED HONEY PEPPER CRUSTED SALMON

This recipe adds a great taste to salmon and takes away any fishy taste. Make sure you read the whole recipe before proceeding because it is a two day procedure. The marinade and the crust are prepared the day before

1 large	salmon steak, 1" thick, skin on sides (any grey skin removed)

Marinade and crust:

1 ½ cups	water
3 tablespoons	coarse salt
1 cup	light brown sugar
1 tablespoon	fresh ginger, peeled and minced
1 teaspoon	crushed bay leaves
1 teaspoon	whole allspice, crushed
1/8 cup	peppercorns, assorted black, pink, green
½ cup	reserved marinade

Combine water, salt, sugar, ginger, bay leaves, and allspice. Bring to a boil. Immediately pour out ½ cup of the liquid and place in bowl. Add peppercorns that have been crushed into very small pieces (I use my coffee grinder, just clean very well before and after use or use a spice grinder) to the ½ cup of liquid. Let steep for 15 minutes and run mixture through a small, fine mesh strainer to strain off the liquid from the peppercorns. What remains in the strainer is a paste that you will use for the crust. Save the liquid that remains to serve on the side with the salmon. After the large quantity of the marinade has cooled to room temperature, pour it over the salmon that has been placed in a small container so that the liquid covers it. Cover and let it marinade overnight. The next morning remove and transfer the salmon to a wire rack with a plate underneath. Discard the marinade. Refrigerate, uncovered, all day until time to prepare for cooking. This procedure is to dry out the exterior surfaces of the salmon.

Preparing the salmon for grilling:

Spread about a tablespoon of honey with the back of a spoon all over the top of the salmon. Then spread the peppercorn paste on top of the honey. Place salmon on foil and grill on low heat, covered grill, until done, will flake with a fork (or you can place salmon in a lightly oiled baking pan and bake in a 350 degree oven until done).

SPICY GRILLED SALMON

½ teaspoon	paprika
½ or 1/4 teaspoon	salt (to taste)
1 or 2 teaspoons	lemon pepper (to taste)
2 teaspoons	light brown sugar
1 teaspoon	garlic salt
1 teaspoon	tarragon
1 teaspoon	basil
	salmon filet

In a small bowl combine paprika, salt, lemon pepper, sugar, garlic, tarragon and basil.
Remove grey skin on salmon and rub seasonings on both sides of filet. Place on foil and grill until flakes.

FRESH TUNA STEAK & SAUCE

If you've ever had fresh tuna, then you know it's nothing like the canned kind! I like to make a little extra to use for tuna salad the next day

1 tablespoon	butter
1 tablespoon	olive or canola oil
2 teaspoons	dried onion flakes
2 teaspoons	garlic, minced
½ teaspoon	ginger
½ cup	dried apricots (without sulfites) finely diced in food processor or by hand
3/4 cup	apple cider vinegar
3/4 cup	apricot juice (or apple juice)
	brown sugar and salt to taste
2	tuna steaks

Heat the oil and butter in small frying pan. Add the onions and garlic and stir until onions are a little brown. Add the ginger and apricots and stir to mix. Add the vinegar, apricot juice, sugar and salt to taste. Simmer on low for a few minutes until sauce thickens.

Grill 2 large tuna steaks according to the "10 Minute Rule" on page 62. Pour sauce over and serve.

Serving Suggestion: Great with baked potato and steamed or grilled veggies

Note: This is a tangy sauce. It you want it a little less tangy, use 1/4 cup of vinegar, ½ cup water, and 3/4 cup apricot juice.

TUNA CASSEROLE

12 ounces	"good" tuna, drained
2	green chilies, de-seeded, roasted, peeled and diced
1	red pepper, de-seeded, roasted, peeled and diced
6 ounces	noodles, (Eden Organic Parsley Garlic Ribbons) cook in boiling water for 1 minute, drain in colander
5 ounces	crushed potato chips (Olive Oil brand chips: Cracked Pepper or Garlic)

White Sauce:

2 tablespoons	butter
2 tablespoons	all purpose flour
1 teaspoon	salt
1/2 teaspoon	pepper, freshly ground
½ teaspoon	paprika
1/4 teaspoon	cayenne
2 ½ cups	milk
1 cup	frozen peas
½ cup	farmer cheese, grated

Melt butter on low heat and stir in flour until smooth and slightly brown. Add salt, pepper, paprika and cayenne. Add milk gradually stirring constantly over medium heat until mixture comes to a boil. Turn down heat and continue to stir until thickens. Mix together sauce, tuna, chiles, red pepper, peas, cheese and pasta. Spoon into an 8" x 8" baking dish and sprinkle crushed potato chips on top. Bake in a 350 degree oven for 30 minutes.

FISH FILET WITH VEGETABLE SAUCE

If you are not overly fond of fish, but want to eat it because it is healthy, this is a tasty way to serve it

1 teaspoon	butter
1 teaspoon	olive oil
2 teaspoons	garlic, minced
2 tablespoons	fresh basil, chopped (or 1 tablespoon dried)
1	red pepper, diced (better if roasted)
2	green chilies, diced (better if roasted)
4	fresh tomatoes, diced
1/4 cup	organic brown rice vinegar
½ teaspoon	salt
2-4	fish filets (mahi mahi, catfish, cod, tuna, snapper, etc.) rubbed with Fish Rub (recipe on page 63)

Heat butter and oil in small frying pan. Add garlic and basil and stir for a minute. Add peppers, chilies and tomatoes. Stir in vinegar and salt. Simmer on low heat while preparing fish.

Heat skillet with enough olive oil to cover bottom of pan. Saute seasoned fish using the "10 minute rule" (page 62) on one side and then the other.

Pour sauce over fish and cover, let rest 5 minutes or you can serve immediately.

GRILLED FISH FILET WITH TANGY SAUCE

2 to 4	fresh fish filets: (halibut, red snapper, or whatever fish you like grilled until flakes
2 teaspoons	canola or olive oil
1/4 cup	dried onion flakes
1 tablespoon	garlic, minced
1 ½ cups	carrots, sliced
1/8 teaspoon	cloves, freshly ground
½ teaspoon	pepper, freshly ground
½ teaspoon	thyme, freshly ground or ½ teaspoon dried marjoram
½ teaspoon	salt
1 cup	chicken stock (recipe on page 33)
2"	cinnamon stick
2-3	green chilies, de-seeded, roasted, peeled and sliced

Heat oil in medium skillet and add onion and garlic. Saute until onions and garlic are lightly browned. Add carrots, cloves, pepper, thyme or marjoram and salt. Stir until well mixed, add stock, and cinnamon stick. Simmer on low for 8-10 minutes and add chilies. Place filets on top of sauce, cover and let sit for a few minutes (up to 30) so the liquid absorbs into the fish. Reheat, if necessary, for a minute or so before serving. You can also serve immediately, pouring sauce over fish.

Serving Suggestion: Great with baked potato

SCALLOPS

6 ounces	noodles (Eden Organic Parsley Garlic Ribbons) cook according to package directions, drain in colander
2 tablespoons	butter
1 teaspoon	roasted garlic oil
1 tablespoon	fresh basil, or ½ tablespoon dried basil
1 teaspoon	garlic, minced
1 pound	large fresh sea scallops salt and pepper to taste

Melt butter, add oil, basil, and garlic. Stir a few times and add scallops, salt and pepper. Saute for 1-2 minutes, until scallops are iridescent. Using tongs, turn and saute on other side for 1-2 minutes more. Don't over cook or they will be tough. Blanch noodles in colander with hot water. Immediately serve scallops and butter sauce over noodles.

Note: Scallops are low in fat and cholesterol. Always buy fresh, rinse, pull off any hard tissue that remains, pat dry before cooking.

LOBSTER TAILS

Bring water to boil in steamer pot. Add tails and steam for 10 minutes. Cut off hard shells with scissors and serve with melted butter.

CURRIED SHRIMP AND RICE

3 tablespoons	butter
1/4 cup	dried onion flakes
1 cup	celery, chopped
1 tablespoon	curry powder
2 tablespoons	flour
1 1/4 cups	milk
1/8 teaspoon	cayenne
½ teaspoon	salt, coarse
1/8 teaspoon	pepper, freshly ground
1 pound	uncooked shrimp, shelled and de-veined

Melt the butter in a medium frying pan. Stir and saute the onions and celery for about a minute or two on medium heat. Stir in the curry. Blend in the flour to form a paste. Add the milk a little a time to avoid lumps. Add cayenne, salt and pepper. Add shrimp and bring to the barely boiling point. Cook for no more than five minutes or until shrimp are cooked through and pink. Serve over rice.

ROGER'S SPICY SHRIMP AND SAUCE

My husband, who is a very creative cook, made this wonderful dish for me

1 tablespoon	rice vinegar
1 cup	apricot or peach juice
2 tablespoons	brown sugar
1/4 teaspoon	tabasco sauce
1/4 teaspoon	salt
1/4 cup	water
2 tablespoons	flour

Mix vinegar, juice, brown sugar, tabasco and salt together in a medium saucepan. In a small bowl mix water and flour until smooth and add to ingredients in pan. Cook and stir until thickened and smooth.

2 tablespoons	butter
½ teaspoon	olive oil
1 teaspoon	basil (dried) or 2 teaspoons fresh
1 teaspoon	garlic, minced
1 large	red pepper, diced
1/8 teaspoon	cayenne
1/8 teaspoon	paprika
1 teaspoon	salt
1 pound	shrimp, raw-shelled and devained

Melt butter and add oil. Add basil, garlic, red pepper, cayenne, paprika, and salt. Saute for a minute until blended. Add shrimp and saute until pink, only takes 1-2 minutes, don't over cook. Add sauce and stir. Serve immediately over cooked wild rice, brown rice or risotto.

SHRIMP AND GARLIC DILL SAUCE

2 tablespoons	butter
1 tablespoon	fresh garlic, minced
1 tablespoon	fresh dill, chopped
2 tablespoons	flour
1 cup	milk (if you want it really rich, use half and half)
½ teaspoon	salt
1 pound	uncooked shrimp, peeled, de-vained and tails removed
	angel hair pasta, cooked according to package directions, drained and blanched in colander. Blanch with hot water before serving

Melt butter in medium frying pan. Add garlic and saute on low heat. Add dill and saute a little more. Add flour and blend until smooth. Add milk very gradually stirring constantly until smooth and hot. Add salt and shrimp and simmer for 2-3 minutes until shrimp are pink and cooked through (don't over-cook or they will be tough).Serve immediately over pasta.

SHRIMP AND SAUCE

3 cups	fresh tomatoes, diced (or 28 ounce can of diced tomatoes)
1 teaspoon	garlic, minced
1 teaspoon	salt
1/4 teaspoon	pepper, freshly ground
1/4 teaspoon	cayenne
1/4 cup	fresh basil, chopped or 1/8 cup dried
1/3 cup	seasoned rice vinegar
1 tablespoon	olive oil
1 tablespoons	butter
1 tablespoon	dried onion flakes
1	yellow or red pepper, finely diced
1 cup	celery, finely diced
1 pound	un-cooked shrimp, peeled, de-veined and tails removed

Mix tomatoes, garlic, salt, pepper, cayenne, basil and vinegar. Set aside.
Heat oil and butter in frying pan and add onion, pepper and celery. Stir a few times until onion is lightly browned. Add sauce and stir until well mixed. Add shrimp and stir. Cook for 2-3 minutes until shrimp is pink and cooked through (don't over-cook or they will be tough).

APPLE SHRIMP

Sauce:

1 tablespoon	butter
½ teaspoon	garlic, minced
2 teaspoons	fresh basil, or 1 teaspoon dried
1/8 teaspoon	cayenne
½ teaspoon	mustard, (recipe on page 129, Rothschild or dry mustard)
1/4 cup	rice vinegar
2 cups	apple juice
1 teaspoon	seasoned rice vinegar
1 teaspoon	honey
2	apples, diced

Melt butter in medium frying pan. Add garlic, basil and cayenne. Stir until well blended. Add mustard, rice vinegar, apple juice, vinegar, honey and apples. Cook on medium high heat until cooked down (about 20 minutes)

1 tablespoon	butter
½ teaspoon	oil
1 cup	carrots, sliced
1 cup	celery, sliced
½ teaspoon	salt
1/4 teaspoon	pepper
1/8 teaspoon	cayenne
1 pound	shrimp, uncooked, peeled, de-veined and tails removed

Heat butter and oil in frying pan or wok. Add carrots, celery, salt, pepper and cayenne. Stir fry for 2-3 minutes (vegetables should still be a little crunchy) and add shrimp. Stir fry for approximately 2-3 minutes or until shrimp is pink (don't over-cook shrimp or they will be tough). Stir in hot sauce and serve immediately. Serve over brown rice, pasta or Couscous (page 91).

MEXICAN DISHES

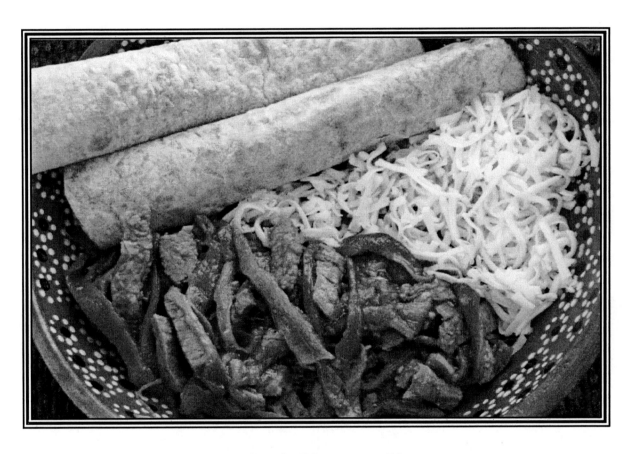

Fajitas for Wayne, page 76

TORTILLAS

These tortillas are very easy to make and so good. If you don't need all of the tortillas at once, you can store the dough balls in the refrigerator for a few days and can even freeze them

4 cups	unbleached white flour
1 teaspoon	salt
1 1/4 cups plus 3 tablespoons	warm water
1/4 cup	canola or olive oil

Mix flour and salt. Add warm water and oil. Knead dough until elastic and smooth, about 5 minutes. Cover and let rest about 15 minutes. Divide dough evenly into 10-12 balls. Working one dough ball at a time, roll out on very lightly floured board into a thin 10 inch circle (can place a piece of plastic wrap on top and on bottom of dough to make rolling out easier). Place rolled out tortillas on a large plate and put a piece of plastic wrap or wax paper between each tortilla. Cook one at a time in a very large hot skillet (to test if hot enough, put a drop of water onto pan, if it immediately evaporates, it is ready). When large bubbles form and tortilla is lightly browned, about a minute, turn (only once). Cook about a minute more or until browned. Be careful not to overcook if you are using it for a burro as you want it to be soft and pliable for rolling. Store on a warm plate covered with a towel until ready to use.

Note: I recently purchased a tortilla press/cooker and it works great!

CHICKEN BURROS

chicken breasts sprinkled with Chicken Rub (recipe on page 33), grilled and cut into thin strips

tortillas (recipe above) or "good" tortillas wrapped in foil and warmed in oven

cheese, grated (Farmer or natural white cheddar)

salsa (recipe on page 73) or Pace Chunky All Natural Salsa

creme fraiche or Daisy sour cream

Lay chicken on one end of warm tortilla, then grated cheese and salsa, top with creme fraiche or sour cream. Fold in sides and roll tortilla.

SALSA

1 tablespoon	garlic oil (Consorzio) or olive or canola oil
1 tablespoon	fresh garlic, minced
2 tablespoons	dried onion flakes
28 ounces	tomatoes (Eden Organic Diced) or fresh, diced
1	red pepper, de-seeded, roasted, peeled and diced
4	green chiles, de-seeded, roasted, peeled and diced
1/8 teaspoon	cumin
1/4 teaspoon	chili powder
1/4 teaspoon	cayenne
1/8 teaspoon	paprika
1 teaspoon	salt

Heat oil on low heat and add garlic and onion. Stir a few times until lightly browned. Add tomatoes, pepper, chilies, cumin, chili powder, cayenne, paprika and salt. Bring to boil and simmer about 30 minutes.

Note: Another version of this recipe is to add 1/4 cup chopped, fresh cilantro and leave out the chilies and red pepper.

TOMATILLO SALSA

10-15	tomatillos, grilled
3	green chilies, de-seeded, roasted, peeled and diced
1	red pepper, de-seeded, roasted, peeled and diced
1/4 cup	packed cilantro leaves
½ teaspoon	lemongrass ginger oil
½ teaspoon	balsamic vinegar
½ teaspoon	salt
1/4 teaspoon	freshly ground pepper
1/8 teaspoon	cayenne

Lay tomatillos, in husks, on a sheet of heavy duty foil in one layer. Place another piece of foil on top and roll the edges tightly. Place on top shelf of grill. Close lid, cook on low, turning once, for about 20-30 minutes (depending on your particular grill). Take off grill and open carefully, pointing away from you. Cool until you can handle. Peel off husks and stems and place in blender or food processor. Add roasted chiles and red pepper, cilantro, oil, vinegar, salt, pepper and cayenne. Blend until smooth.

Note: Makes 4 cups

Serving Suggestion: Great on cheese crisp, or for dip

CREAM CHEESE CHICKEN ENCHILADAS

3 cups	finely chopped grilled chicken (4 chicken breasts rubbed with Chicken Rub (recipe on page 33) and grilled
3 or 4	green chilies, de-seeded, roasted, peeled and diced
8	tortillas (recipe on page 72 or "good" tortillas)
3-4 cups	salsa (recipe on page 73 or Pace Chunky)
	grated farmer cheese (optional)

Filling:

1 teaspoon	olive or canola oil
½ cup	dried onion flakes
12 ounces	(1 ½ cups) cream cheese (Gina Marie)
1 ½ cups	milk
3/4 teaspoon	salt (or to taste)

Heat oil in small frying pan, add onions and saute until golden brown. Add cream cheese and stir constantly until cheese is melted and smooth. Add milk and salt and continue to stir constantly until mixture is creamy and thickened. Add chopped grilled chicken and chilies. Heat tortillas in oven, wrapped in foil (if they are very soft, no need to heat first). Spread 2-3 tablespoons filling on one end of tortilla (not all the way to edge), fold in sides and roll up. Place in lightly oiled 9" x 13" baking pan, seam side down. Pour salsa over, cover with foil and bake in a 350 degree oven for approximately 20 minutes, uncover and sprinkle with cheese and bake for 5 more minutes.

Note: This filling is also very good to put in a heated tortilla without the sauce.

TORTILLA CHIP CASSEROLE

4 cups	tortilla chips, broken a little (Padrino's or Guiltless Gourmet)
4	chicken breasts sprinkled with Chicken Rub (recipe on page 33) grilled and diced or use boiled chicken pieces
2-24 ounce jars	salsa, Pace Chunky or salsa recipe on page 73
2-8 ounce	creme fraiche (Vermont Butter and Cheese Company) or Daisy sour cream
1 ½ cups	farmer cheese, grated
1 ½ cups	natural white cheddar cheese, grated

Place 2 cups of tortilla chips in the bottom of a 8" x 13" baking pan. Place half of the diced chicken on top of the chips and cover with half of the salsa. Spoon 1 cup of the creme fraiche on top of salsa and top with half of both cheeses. Repeat layers topping with grated cheese. Bake in a 375 degree oven for 30-40 minutes until bubbling. Let set for 5 minutes before cutting.

Note: For a smaller version of this recipe, half the ingredients for only one layer and use an 8" x 11" pan.

BEEF BURROS

2 pounds	thinly sliced round steak or flank steak cut in bite size pieces
1 tablespoon	garlic oil
1 tablespoon	garlic, minced
1/8 teaspoon	cayenne
1/8 teaspoon	cumin
2 tablespoons	cilantro (fresh) or 1 tablespoon dried
½ teaspoon	salt
1- 1 ½ cups	salsa (recipe on page 73 or Pace Chunky)
1	red pepper, de-seeded, roasted, peeled and thinly sliced
1	yellow pepper, de-seeded, roasted, peeled and thinly sliced
1	green pepper, de-seeded, roasted, peeled and thinly sliced
2	green chilies, de-seeded, roasted, peeled and thinly sliced
	grated farmer or natural cheddar cheese
8-10	warm tortillas (recipe on page 72 or "good" tortillas)

Heat garlic oil over medium heat. Add meat and stir fry until brown. Add minced garlic, cayenne, cumin, cilantro (if using fresh, add later with the salsa), and salt. Add ½ cup water, cover and simmer for 1-1 ½ hours or until tender. Check often and add water as needed, ½ cup at a time. When tender remove lid and simmer until most of the liquid is gone. Add salsa and simmer for a few more minutes. Add peppers, chilies and onions. Lay meat mixture on one end of warm tortilla, sprinkle with cheese, fold in sides and roll up.

Note: You can also do the meat mixture in a slow cooker. Add the salsa, peppers, chilies and onions the last 20 minutes.

GREEN CHILI

4 pounds	lean stew meat or cut up roast in bite size pieces, fat cut off
1 tablespoon	minced garlic
½ cup	dried onion flakes
1 tablespoon	chili powder
1 teaspoon	oregano
1 teaspoon	cumin
½ teaspoon	crushed red pepper
½ teaspoon	cayenne
4 teaspoons	salt
1 teaspoon	pepper
2 cups	green chiles, de-seeded, roasted, peeled and diced
5 - 28 ounce	crushed tomatoes, or fresh blended tomatoes
12 ounces	tomato paste
large	tortillas, (recipe on page 72 or "good" tortillas)
	grated cheese (if desired)

Put flour in zipper bag and shake meat until coated. Place meat in large wire strainer and shake over sink or bowl until excess flour is gone. Heat oil (enough to cover bottom of pot) in large cooker and cook meat, stirring often (one layer of meat at a time) until brown and oil is gone. Add garlic and onions and stir a few times. Add the chili powder, oregano, red pepper, cayenne, salt and pepper. Stir until well blended, then add the tomatoes. Simmer for a couple of hours until meat is very tender and sauce is thickened.

Place a large spoonful of chile on one end of tortilla, sprinkle cheese on top, fold in sides and roll.

FAJITAS FOR WAYNE

My son loves fajitas, so after several tries, I came up with this recipe which he loves!

1 tablespoon	olive or canola oil
1 tablespoon	garlic, minced
1/4 teaspoon	crushed red pepper
½ teaspoon	salt
1 ½ pound	flank steak, cut in thin bite sized strips across the grain on a slight diagonal

Heat oil in a large frying pan or wok. Add garlic, red pepper, salt and stir. Add steak strips and stir fry until brown. Simmer on low heat, covered, until all the liquid is gone, about 30 minutes. Check often so it won't cook dry. If it isn't as tender as you want, add a little water and continue to simmer until tender. Take the steak out, put on a plate and cover to keep warm.

1	red pepper, de-seeded and cut in thin slices
1	green pepper, de-seeded and cut in thin slices
1	yellow pepper, de-seeded and cut in thin slices
4	green chilies, de-seeded, roasted, peeled and thin sliced
	grated farmer or white cheddar cheese

Add a little oil to pan and add sliced peppers to wok. Stir fry until brown and a little tender.

8	tortillas (recipe on page 72)
	salsa (recipe on page 73 or Pace Chunky)

Lay meat, peppers and chilies on tortilla. Top with a little salsa and grated cheese, fold in sides and roll up.

Note:　　　　　You can also make recipe with chicken.

CHICKEN TORTILLA CASSEROLE

1 large	whole chicken (or 2 small), boiled, cooled, pulled apart and diced (6 cups) or 6 grilled chicken breasts, seasoned with Chicken Rub (recipe on page 33) and diced
8	green chiles, de-seeded, roasted, peeled and sliced or two 8 ounce cans
7 cups	fresh tomatoes, blended, or two 28 ounce cans crushed tomatoes
½ cup	dried onion flakes
1 tablespoon	garlic, minced
2 teaspoons	salt
1 teaspoon	Spice Hunter Fajita Seasoning (or your own combination of spices)
2 tablespoons	fresh cilantro, chopped or 1 tablespoon dried
1 dozen	corn tortillas, cut in half twice
16 ounces	farmers cheese (solid), grated
1 ½ cups	milk or half and half

Bring chicken to a boil in very large pot and cook on low boil for about 1 ½-2 hours. Turn once or twice (while chicken is cooking make sauce and roast chilies).

Take chicken out of water and place on platter or cookie sheet. Pull apart with forks to allow the chicken to cool faster. Separate "good" meat and throw away the rest. Cut chicken into small pieces.

Pour tomatoes into saucepan, add the onions, garlic, salt, seasoning and cilantro. Bring to a boil and simmer for about 30 minutes or until thickened.

With scissors, cut tortillas in half and then cut them in half again. Spray a little oil on the bottom of an 8" x 12" baking pan and lay half of the cut tortillas on the bottom of the pan, then half of the cut up chicken, half of the green chiles, half of the cheese, half of the sauce, half of the milk. Layer again starting with the cut tortillas and ending with the milk.

Bake in a 350 degree oven for 50 minutes or until it looks pretty firm and bubbling. Let set for 5 minutes before cutting.

Note: This recipe makes a lot. Cut recipe in half for 4-6 people.

PASTA DISHES

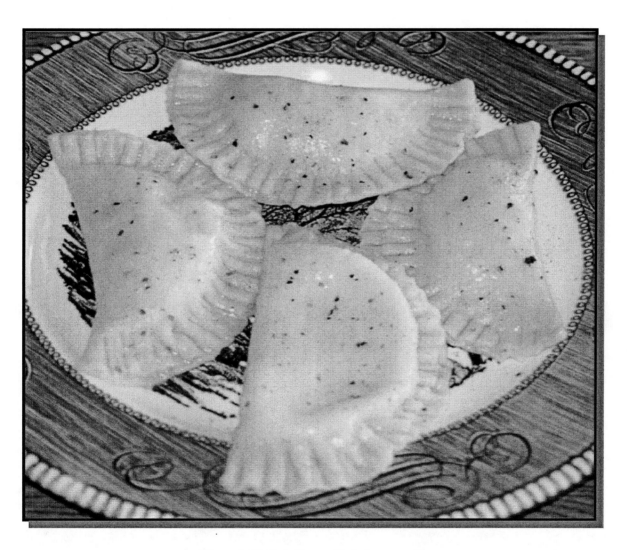

Pierogi (Polish Dumplings), page 82

PASTA TIPS

1. For every pound of pasta, boil in 5 quarts of water

2. Pasta will cook a little more after taking out of boiling water. Make sure it is a little firmer than what you want.

3. Pour pasta immediately into colander in the sink and rinse with cool water to stop it cooking and to remove starch.

4. Add a tablespoon of butter to the water to keep it from boiling over and to keep it from sticking together. Cover the pot, bring to a boil and add salt and the pasta after the water boils. Uncover and cook until "al dente".

5. For chunky sauce, use dense pasta (penne, bows, etc.). For smooth sauce, use angel hair, thin spaghetti, etc.

SPAGHETTI

2 pounds	lean ground sirloin, lean ground beef or ground turkey
2 tablespoons	dried onion flakes
2 tablespoons	garlic, minced
4 tablespoons	fresh oregano (2 tablespoons dried)
4 tablespoons	fresh basil (2 tablespoons dried)
1 ½ tablespoons	salt
½ teaspoon	cumin
1 teaspoon	cayenne
1/4 teaspoon	paprika
1 teaspoon	chili powder
1 teaspoon	onion powder
4 - 28 ounce cans	tomatoes (diced or crushed Eden Organic) or approximately 13 organic (if possible) very large tomatoes (blended, leaving some chunks) making 14 cups
12 ounce	tomato paste
	cooked pasta (DeBoles Organic Whole Wheat Pasta)

In medium frying pan, brown beef and drain off any excess fat (if you want to remove all fat from beef, rinse in colander with cold water and return to frying pan). Stir and mix into beef, onion, garlic, oregano, basil, salt, cumin, cayenne, paprika, chili powder, and onion powder. Add tomatoes and paste and mix well. Cover and simmer on low, just so its bubbling a little, for about 2-4 hours stirring occasionally.

Serving Suggestion: Sprinkle a little grated farmer cheese on top. Garlic french bread or homemade bread and a salad are perfect with this dish.

Menu Planning Tip: Freeze some of the sauce for another meal such as: manicotti, lasagna, pierogi or pizza. Be sure you label, date, and write amount on container.

LASAGNA

15	lasagna noodles
30 ounces	ricotta cheese (Polly O Original)
16 ounces	fresh mozzarella
24 ounces	farmer cheese (may bud)

Sauce: (or 9 cups of leftover spaghetti sauce)

1 ½ pounds	ground sirloin or very lean ground beef
1 ½ tablespoons	onion flakes
1 ½ tablespoons	garlic, minced
3 tablespoons	fresh oregano or 1 ½ tablespoons dried oregano
3 tablespoons	fresh basil or 1 ½ tablespoons dried basil
1 tablespoon	salt
½ teaspoon	cumin
½ teaspoon	cayenne
1/4 teaspoon	paprika
3/4 teaspoon	chile powder
3/4 teaspoon	onion powder
3 - 28 ounce cans	tomatoes (Eden Organic)
12 ounce can	tomato paste

In medium frying pan brown beef and drain off any excess fat (if you want to remove all the fat from beef, rinse in colander with cold water and return to frying pan). Add onion, garlic, oregano, basil, salt, cumin, cayenne, paprika, chile powder, onion powder. Stir and mix well with beef. Add tomatoes and tomato paste and mix well. Cover and simmer on low, just so it is bubbling a little for two to four hours, stirring occasionally.

Cook noodles in boiling salted water for four minutes, just until pliable. Dump into a colander in the sink and rinse with cold water. Immediately lay the noodles flat on waxed paper on the counter. Put a 1 ½ cups of sauce to cover the bottom of a 9" x 13" pan and lay four noodles lengthwise and one across. Put 2 ½ cups of sauce on top of noodles. Mix all the cheeses together (10 cups) and put 3 cups of it on top of sauce. Layer two more times ending with cheese. Bake in a 375 degree oven for 45 minutes to one hour, until bubbly and hot. Let set for 10 minutes (will cut better).

MANICOTTI

2 cups	fresh spinach (optional)
2 teaspoons	canola oil
½ teaspoon	salt
½ teaspoon	pepper
1/8 teaspoon	nutmeg
½ teaspoon	oregano
15 ounces	ricotta cheese (Polly O Original)
8 ounces	grated fresh mozzarella (will make 2 cups)
2 ounces	grated farmer cheese (will make ½ cup)
1	egg, slightly beaten
3-4 cups	Spaghetti sauce (recipe on page 79)
14	manicotti pasta tubes. Place in boiling water for 5 minutes and immediately rinse with cold water in colander. Then place on waxed paper in single layer

Compact spinach leaves in measuring cup to measure 2 cups (cooks down to 1/4 cup).Wash spinach leaves thoroughly and chop finely. Saute spinach with oil until dry and add salt, pepper, nutmeg and oregano. Place in refrigerator for about 15 minutes until cool. Mix spinach with ricotta, mozzarella, farmer cheese and egg. Stir until very well blended (if you don't use spinach, add the salt, pepper, nutmeg, and oregano to the cheese and egg mixture)

Fill cooked manicotti tubes using a pastry bag or a cake decorating tube with a large tip. The easiest way to do this is to stand the manicotti up in a coffee mug or short glass and fill one end and then the other. Spread a little sauce to cover the bottom of a 9" x 13" baking pan and place manicotti side by side. Pour the rest of the sauce over the tubes and cover with foil. Can grate a little farmer cheese on top. Bake in a 350 degree oven for 30-40 minutes until heated through.

Serving Suggestion: Serve Honey Oatmeal Bread (recipe on page 120) or "good" garlic bread and a salad.

Note: Instead of using manicotti shells, you can also use 8 ounces of noodles (Eden Organic Garlic Ribbons). Spray 8" x 8" pan with a little oil. Layer half of noodles (Place in boiling water and boil for only 1 minute and drain), then half of cheese mixture, remaining noodles and remaining cheese. Pour 2 cups of sauce on top. Bake for 20-30 minutes until hot and bubbling.

PIEROGI (Polish Dumplings)

Dough:

1	egg
1 tablespoon	creme fraiche (Vermont Butter and Cream Co.) or sour cream (Daisy)
½ cup	milk
½ cup	water
2 1/4 - 2 ½ cups	unbleached all purpose flour

In a medium bowl, whisk egg. Add creme fraiche or sour cream and whisk until smooth. Add the milk and water and whisk until combined. Slowly add 2 cups of flour and stir to combine. Place dough on a floured surface and work in about 1/4 cup of flour as you knead. Use a plastic scraper to lift the dough which will stick to the cutting board or counter before the flour is worked into it. Continue kneading for about 6-8 minute working in a little more flour if needed. The dough should be elastic in texture and no longer sticky. Be careful not to add too much flour, as this will toughen dough. Form into a ball and place an inverted bowl over it. Let dough rest under bowl for 15 minutes. Divide the dough in half. On a large floured cutting board, roll dough out until very thin. Using a 3" cookie cutter or glass, cut out circles (will make 21). Gather scraps, re-roll and continue cutting. In a rounded tablespoon, form filling into a ball and place in the center of each dough circle. Holding the circle in your hand, fold dough over filling and pinch the edges together forming a well sealed crescent. Transfer each crescent to a linen towel. Cover with another linen towel. Place pierogi in about 4 quarts of boiling water in batches. After water starts to boil again, cook for a minute for a total of 3 minutes. Take out with slotted spoon and place in single layer on platter. Serve immediately, with sauce (spaghetti sauce, cream sauce or just melted butter with salt and freshly ground pepper).

Filling:

8 ounces	finely grated farmer cheese
	salt and pepper to taste

Or:

4 pounds	green cabbage, trimmed and cored
8 ounces	cream cheese (Gina Marie) room temperature
2 tablespoons	butter, melted
1 teaspoon	salt
1 ½ teaspoons	pepper

Cut the cabbage into quarters. Steam until very tender, about 20 to 30 minutes, drain and cool. Working in small batches, wrap cooled cabbage in towel and squeeze out as much liquid as possible (you'll use lots of towels). Chop squeezed cabbage finely by hand or in a food processor. Place in bowl and add cream cheese, 4 tablespoons of melted butter and salt and pepper to taste. Mix until well combined. The filling can be made the day ahead if it is kept tightly covered and refrigerated. Serve with melted butter.

Note:	Use the dough the same day. Is hard to work with after being refrigerated. If you do want some for the next day, make them into pierogi's, wrap well, all you'll have to do is boil them.

CREAMY TOMATO CHICKEN & PEAS

4	boneless, skinless chicken breasts cut in bite sized pieces
2 tablespoons	butter
1 tablespoon	canola or olive oil
2 tablespoons	fresh basil (1 tablespoon dried basil)
2 teaspoons	garlic, minced
1 teaspoon	salt, coarse
½ teaspoon	pepper, freshly ground
28 ounces	diced tomatoes (Eden Organic) or fresh
1 cup	milk (or if you like richer, use ½ & ½ or cream)
1 cup	frozen peas

Heat butter and oil in large frying pan. Stir in basil, garlic, salt and pepper until well blended. Add chicken pieces. Stir and saute over medium heat until browned. Add tomatoes and simmer for 20 minutes. Add milk and simmer on low for 10 more minutes. Stir in peas until hot, about 5 more minutes. Serve with pasta.

PASTA AND SAUCE

1 tablespoon	canola or olive oil
2 teaspoons	garlic, minced
2 tablespoons	fresh basil (or 1 tablespoon dried)
1/4 cup	dried onion flakes
14 ounces	fresh diced tomatoes or canned (Eden Organic)
1 teaspoon	salt, coarse
½ teaspoon	pepper, freshly ground
½ cup	milk (use cream or half and half if you want richer)
½ cup	farmer cheese, grated
2 cups	spiral or penne pasta, cooked according to package directions

Heat oil in medium frying pan and add garlic, basil and onion. Saute for a minute or so. Add tomatoes and salt and pepper. Stir and simmer for 5 minutes on medium low heat. Add milk and cheese and stir until well blended and cheese is melted and mixture is hot. Serve immediately over penne pasta. Grate a little cheese on each serving.

ROASTED ZUCCHINI PASTA

4 medium	zucchini's
1 teaspoon	butter
1 teaspoon	canola or garlic oil
1 teaspoon	garlic, minced
1/4 cup	parsley, fresh, chopped (or 1/8 cup dried)
1/4 cup	basil, fresh, chopped (or 1/8 cup dried)
2 tablespoons	butter
2 tablespoons	unbleached all purpose flour
½ teaspoon	salt, coarse
½ teaspoon	pepper, freshly ground
1 - 1 1/4 cup	milk
1/2 cup	farmer cheese, grated
4 ounce jar	"good" pimentos
8 ounces	angel hair pasta (cooked according to package directions)

Scrub zucchini's, cut off ends and slice evenly (approximately 1/4" slices). Place slices in one layer on lightly oiled, parchment or Silpat lined cookie sheet. Place rack in upper part of oven and broil until light brown, turn over and broil until light brown on other side.

Melt butter with oil in medium frying pan. Saute garlic, parsley and basil for a minute. In same pan, melt 2 more tablespoons butter. Add flour and stir constantly over low heat until smooth. Add salt and pepper. Gradually add milk stirring constantly until thickened and smooth. Add more milk as needed to make the right consistency (you don't want it too thick, but not too thin). Add cheese and pimentos and stir until cheese is melted. Place portion of pasta on plate, top with zucchini and spoon sauce over.

MACARONI AND CHEESE

2 3/4 cups	milk
3 tablespoons	butter
1/4 cup	flour
3/4 teaspoon	salt
1/2 teaspoon	freshly ground pepper
1/8 teaspoon	freshly ground nutmeg
1/8-1/4 teaspoon	cayenne
8 ounces	natural, white cheddar cheese, grated (makes 2 1/4 cups)
2 cups	elbow macaroni, uncooked
1 cup	finely processed "good" bread crumbs
1 tablespoon	butter, melted

Heat the milk in a medium saucepan, but do not boil. In another medium saucepan, over low heat, melt the 3 tablespoons of butter. When butter is melted, stir or whisk in the flour until smooth. Add the milk, a little at a time, stirring constantly over medium heat until mixture is thick and bubbling. Remove from heat and stir in salt, pepper, nutmeg, cayenne and cheese.
While bringing 3 quarts of water to a boil, mix bread crumbs with melted butter and butter a 1 ½ quart baking dish. Add the macaroni to boiling water and boil for 3 minutes (less than directions on package, you want it to be very firm so it won't overcook in the oven). Drain in colander and rinse with cold water. Drain well and add to cheese sauce. Pour mixture into buttered pan and sprinkle on bread crumb mixture. Bake, covered, in a 350 degree oven for 20 minutes. Uncover and bake for 5 more minutes until browned on top.

EGGPLANT PENNE PASTA

1	eggplant
	kosher salt
1 tablespoon	canola or olive oil
1 tablespoon	minced garlic
2 tablespoons	fresh basil (or 1 tablespoon dried)
28 ounces	diced tomatoes (Eden Organic)
1 teaspoon	salt, coarse
½ teaspoon	pepper, freshly ground
8 ounces	penne pasta
	grated farmer or mozzarella cheese

Peel eggplant and cut in half lengthwise, cut in half again and cut into bite sized pieces about 1/2". Place one layer on plate, sprinkle with salt, another layer and salt again. Let set for 30 minutes while you prepare the sauce. This process takes out the bitterness.

Heat oil in saucepan and add garlic. Stir a few times over low heat and add basil. Stir. Add tomatoes, salt and pepper. Let simmer on low heat while you prepare the eggplant and pasta.

In a 10"-11" skillet add 1 ½ cups oil. Throughly rinse eggplant in a colander. Place the drained eggplant on large clean dishtowel and pat dry. When the oil is very hot, add some of the eggplant and cook until light brown on each side. Using a slotted spoon transfer the eggplant to paper towel lined plate. Cook the rest of the eggplant.

Bring salted water to a boil and add pasta. Cook for about 10-12 minutes (until al dente). Drain pasta, place in a large bowl and pour sauce over and mix well. Add the eggplant. Grate cheese over each portion.

CHEESY BEEF AND NOODLE CASSEROLE

1 pound	ground sirloin (or very lean ground beef)
1/4 cup	dried onion flakes
1 tablespoon	dried oregano (or 2 tablespoons fresh, chopped)
1/8 teaspoon	cayenne
1 teaspoon	salt
1 teaspoon	garlic, minced
6 ounces	tomato paste (Muir Glen, Contadina)
1 cup	water
8 ounces	noodles (Eden Organic Parsley Ribbons) boil for 3 minutes, drain in colander
1 cup	creme fraiche (Vermont Butter and Cheese Co.) or sour cream (Daisy)
1 cup	cottage cheese (Alta Dena Farmer Style) or ricotta (Polly O Original)
1 cup	farmer cheese, grated (may-bud)

Saute beef until brown. Drain off any excess liquid. Add onion, oregano, cayenne, salt and garlic. Stir in tomato paste and add water. Simmer for 20 minutes stirring occasionally until thickened.

Combine cooked and drained noodles with creme fraiche or sour cream. Lightly oil a 9" x 9" casserole dish. Spoon in half of the meat mixture, then half of the noodle mixture, all of the cottage cheese, half of the farmer cheese, the rest of the meat mixture, the rest of the noodle mixture, and top with the rest of the farmer cheese. Cover with foil and bake in a 350 degree oven for 40 minutes. Let sit for 7 minutes before cutting.

STEAK AND SHRIMP STIR FRY

1 tablespoon	olive or canola oil
1 tablespoon	garlic, minced
1/4 teaspoon	crushed red pepper
½ teaspoon	salt
1- 1 ½ pound	flank steak, cut across the grain, diagonally, in thin bite size strips

Sauce:

½ cup	apricot juice
1/4 cup	brown sugar
1 tablespoon	cranberry ginger balsamic vinegar (Wild Thymes)
1 tablespoon	rice vinegar
dash	tabasco sauce
1 tablespoon	flour
1 cup	celery, sliced
1 cup	leeks, upper white part, sliced
1 cup	cabbage, shredded
½ pound	uncooked jumbo shrimp (about 9 or 10) peeled and de-veined
8 ounces	pasta, cooked according to package directions, rinsed with cool water in colander (angel hair, broken in half)

Heat oil in wok or large frying pan. Add garlic, red pepper and salt. Stir a few times and add steak strips and stir fry until brown. Simmer, on low heat, covered, until all the liquid is gone, about 30 minutes. Check often so it won't cook dry. If it is not as tender as you want, add a little water and continue to simmer. While steak is simmering, mix the apricot juice, sugar, vinegars, tabasco sauce and flour in a small saucepan and stir until smooth. Simmer over low heat until hot and thickened. Prepare vegetables. When steak is done, remove from pan. Add a little oil if none is left in pan and when pan is very hot, stir fry celery, leeks, and cabbage for about 2 minutes, you want the vegetables to be crunchy. Add the shrimp, steak and sauce and stir until shrimp is pink and cooked through (only takes 2-3 minutes, don't overcook). Serve immediately over the cooked pasta or it's good all by itself.

FRESH HERB PASTA

You can use dried herbs, but fresh tastes SO much better! This makes a great lunch or a light dinner for 2-3 people

1 tablespoon	lemongrass ginger oil
½ cup	canola or olive oil
2 tablespoons	rice vinegar
1 large	garlic clove, peeled and cut up
1 cup (packed)	parsley leaves, fresh (or ½ cup dried)
1 tablespoon	mint leaves, fresh (or ½ tablespoon dried)
1 tablespoon	marjoram leaves, fresh (or ½ tablespoon dried leaves or 1 teaspoon powdered)
1 tablespoon	thyme leaves, fresh (or ½ tablespoon dried leaves or ½ teaspoon powdered)
3/4 -1 teaspoon	salt
½ teaspoon	pepper
2 cups	asparagus (thin) fresh, cut in bite sized pieces (or broccoli or half of each)
2 cups	cherry tomatoes, cut in half or diced tomatoes
½ cup - 1 cup	farmer cheese, grated
2 cups	bow tie pasta
1 tablespoon	salt

In a food processor or blender place the oils, vinegar, garlic, parsley, mint, marjoram, thyme, salt and pepper. Process until smooth and pour sauce into small saucepan.

Steam the cut up asparagus for 2-3 minutes. Drain and place rinse in cold water.

Place pasta and 1 tablespoon of salt in boiling water and cook for 8-10 minutes after water comes back to boil. Drain in colander and rinse with cool water.

Heat sauce. In large bowl, combine the pasta, sauce, asparagus, tomatoes, and cheese and stir to combine. Serve immediately.

Note: This salad tastes great warm or cold. Store any leftovers in the refrigerator.

EGG DISHES

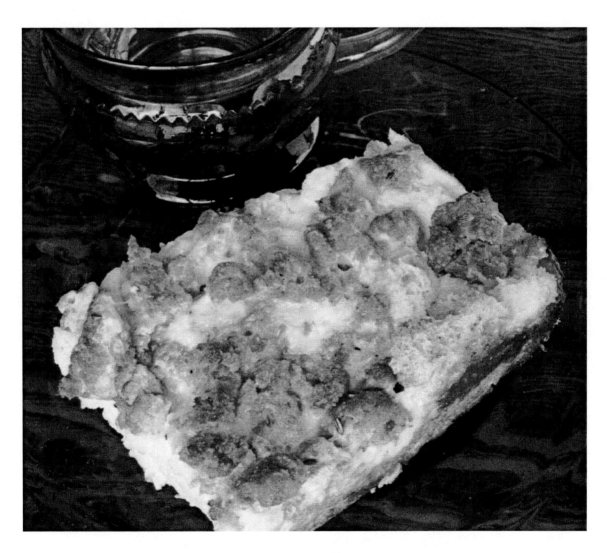

Egg and Sausage Souffle, page 90

QUICHE

Crust:

2 cups	all purpose flour
½ cup (1 stick)	butter
1/8 teaspoon	salt
½ cup	ice water (may need more or less, add water gradually until right consistency)

Cut small pieces of butter into flour, add salt. Using pastry blender or fork, cut in butter until crumbly. Add cold water. Form into a ball & place on floured board. (For flaky crust, try not to handle too much). Roll out in a large circle. Place rolling pin on one end of dough, roll dough around rolling pin. Lay dough in 9" pie plate. Cut dough around edge leaving about 1/2". Fold dough under and crimp by placing both index fingers on dough and pushing together to form a crimp. Prick bottom and sides with fork. Partially bake in a 400 degree oven for 5 minutes.

Filling:

8 ounces	fresh mozzarella, grated or 8 ounces farmer cheese, grated
1 ½ cup	broccoli cut up very small (or other fresh veggies)
	Lay grated cheese and broccoli on bottom of pie crust, grind a little nutmeg, S&P and chopped fresh basil on top or whatever seasonings you like

Custard:

3	eggs
2 tablespoons	flour
½ teaspoon	salt
½ teaspoon	white pepper
1/4 teaspoon	paprika
1/8 teaspoon	cayenne
1 ½ cups	half and half (or can use 1 cup heavy cream, & ½ cup milk) (Land of Lakes, Horizon, Alta Dena)

Whisk eggs and then add flour, salt, pepper, paprika, cayenne and half and half until well mixed. Pour custard into prepared crust and bake in a 350 degree oven for 45-55 minutes or until toothpick comes out clean. Let quiche rest for 8 minutes before slicing.

Note: For seafood quiche use: ½ cup (approximately ½ pound) cooked snow crab claws, meat taken out and cut up, ½ cup (approximately ½ pound) cooked shrimp, cut up, and ½ cup (approximately ½ pound) cooked salmon, cut up. Add to custard and put into crust and bake according to directions. You can use lots of other fish variations, chicken or any other vegetables (if you are using high moisture vegetables such as zucchini, or tomatoes, they should be cooked first to evaporate some of their water).

Serving Suggestion: Great with fresh fruit

EGG WHITE OMELET

This is a wonderful alternative to a high fat omelet and it is so good. I really prefer this over the traditional kind. Make sure you have all your ingredients ready before you start cooking. A two sided omelet pan is really essential and is very inexpensive, found at most kitchen stores

4-6	egg whites (room temperature)
1/4 teaspoon	salt and pepper or to taste
1/4 teaspoon	mustard (recipe on page 129, Rothschild or dry mustard)
1/8 teaspoon	paprika
½ cup	diced fresh tomatoes, roasted red pepper, chiles (other veggies)
1-2 teaspoons	fresh herbs (basil, oregano, cilantro)
½ cup	farmer cheese, natural cheddar, or fresh mozzarella
1-2 teaspoons	butter

These amounts are approximate, you have to experiment to find the amounts and ingredients you like.

Omelet pan recipe:

Whisk egg whites until foamy and a little stiff, add seasonings. Melt butter on both sides of pan until it sizzles, but don't let it brown. Pour half of egg white mixture in each side of omelet pan. When it starts to cook a little on edges, lay veggies and cheese on top of eggs on one side. Let it cook a little more until set and flip lid over. Cook approximately 3 minutes on each side (if toothpick comes out clean, it's done)

8" no stick fry pan method:

Heat butter in pan. Pour eggs or egg whites into hot skillet. Over high heat, quickly shake skillet while cooking until eggs are set. Using a spatula, pull eggs away from side of pan to allow uncooked eggs to set. Put ingredients (cheese, tomatoes, chilis, etc) on one side of eggs. When you can easily lift up the other side, fold it over. Lower heat and cover pan until eggs are done.

Note:	Egg whites have 3.5 grams of protein, 0 fat, 0 carbs
	Whole eggs have 70% fat 6.9 grams, 6.2 grams protein, 0 carbs
Note:	Sometimes, I save the egg yolks for Baked Custard (recipe on page 143). Use within a day or two.

FRENCH TOAST

1 pint	fresh strawberries
	sugar
2 large	eggs
1/4 cup	milk
1/8 teaspoon	cinnamon
½ teaspoon	vanilla
4 slices	Cinnamon Bread (recipe on page 121)

Wash and cut up strawberries. Mix with a little sugar. Set aside. Whisk the eggs, milk, cinnamon, and vanilla. Dip each slice of bread into the egg mixture to coat on both sides. Place slices on plate. Butter a griddle and cook each slice until well browned on both sides. Serve with strawberries and juice.

BREAKFAST EGG TORTILLAS
These are great to make when you go camping

1 dozen	eggs
1 teaspoon	salt, coarse
½ teaspoon	pepper, freshly ground
1/8 teaspoon	cayenne
1/8 teaspoon	paprika
1 teaspoon	butter
3	green chiles, de-seeded, roasted, peeled, and diced
1 roasted	red pepper, de-seeded, roasted, peeled, and diced
1 large	tomato, chopped
½ cup	farmer cheese, grated
8	tortillas (recipe on page 72) wrapped in foil and heated in oven (or you can heat individually in frying pan or on burner)

Whisk eggs, add salt, pepper, cayenne and paprika. Melt butter in frying pan. Add egg mixture, chilies, pepper, tomato, and cheese. Stir until eggs are set but still moist. Spoon eggs on one end of tortilla, fold in ends and roll up.

EGG AND SAUSAGE SOUFFLE

½ pound	sausage (recipe on page 61, Hans or Golden Farms Mild Italian Sausage)
2 cups	cubed bread
1 cup	natural white cheddar or farmer cheese, grated
5	eggs, slightly beaten
2 cups	milk
½ teaspoon	dry mustard
½ teaspoon	salt
1/4 teaspoon	pepper, freshly ground
1/8 teaspoon	onion powder
1/8 teaspoon	paprika

Brown sausage. Put through strainer to drain off fat, cool and crumble. Place bread in an 8" x 8" buttered baking pan. Sprinkle with cheese and sausage. Mix the eggs, milk, mustard, salt, pepper, onion powder and paprika. Cover tightly and refrigerate overnight. Bake uncovered in a 325 degree oven for 40-50 minutes or until knife comes out clean. Let set for 5 minutes before cutting. Serves 4.

Serving Suggestion: Great with fruit

SIDE DISHES

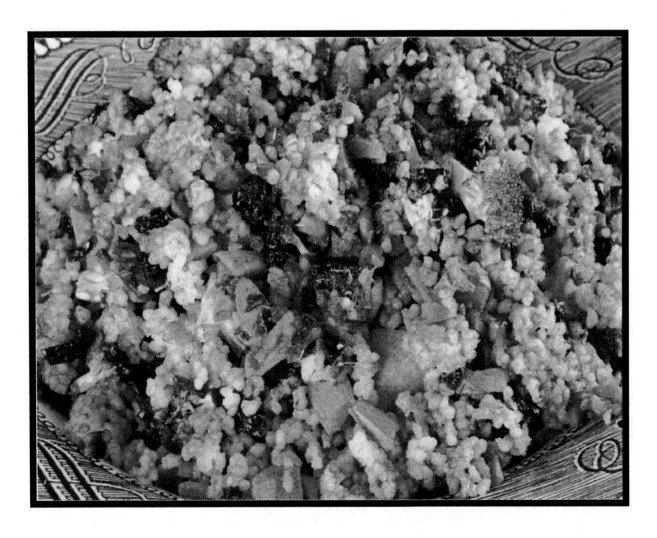

Couscous, page 91

LORI'S SPICY SWEET PEPPER RICE

My daughter Lori, who is a great, healthy cook, made this for us. It is a great way to make the usual bland tasting rice taste great

1 teaspoon	salt
½ teaspoon	onion powder
½ teaspoon	garlic powder
½ teaspoon	pepper, freshly ground
1/8 teaspoon	cayenne
½ teaspoon	dry mustard
½ teaspoon	sage (1 teaspoon fresh)
1/4 teaspoon	nutmeg
1/4 teaspoon	white pepper

Mix above ingredients in small bowl and set aside.

1 small	red pepper, de-seeded and finely diced (roasted is best)
1 small	yellow or green pepper, de-seeded and finely diced (roasted is best)
1/4 cup	apple juice
1 cup	brown rice
2 cups	chicken stock (recipe on page 33)

Lightly spray a medium size frying pan with a little oil. When oil is hot, add diced peppers. Stir and saute for a minute. Add the seasonings (mixed above) and apple juice. Stir to mix. Add the rice and stock. Cover, bring to a boil and simmer on low for about 40 minutes or until liquid is absorbed and rice is tender. (Be sure to cook on low because the rice will need the 40 minutes to get tender. Check occasionally to make sure the liquid is not being absorbed to fast. Add more stock or water if needed.

COUSCOUS

I was really excited when I found this product! Couscous grain is a totally natural product made of pure durum wheat semolina. Make sure the brand you buy does not contain additives, most don't if you buy "plain". It is low in cholesterol. It is very versatile as a side dish, you can add anything you like to it, different herbs, spices, vegetables or even fruit

½ cup	sun dried tomatoes (no sulfur dioxide) or recipe on page 22
1 tablespoon	butter
1 teaspoon	garlic, minced
1 cup	broccoli tops, finely diced
1 cup	carrots, peeled and finely diced
	couscous cooked according to directions for 4 servings (Rivoire Carret is a great brand)

Place sun dried tomatoes in small bowl and add boiling water just to cover. Let sit for 10 minutes. Cook couscous according to package directions. Take tomatoes out of water and finely dice. Reserve ½ cup water. Heat butter in small frying pan. Add garlic, tomatoes, broccoli, and carrots and stir for a minute or two. Add reserved liquid from tomatoes. Stir vegetable mixture into couscous and serve.

RISOTTO/SPANISH RICE

1 teaspoon	olive oil
1 teaspoon	butter
1 tablespoon	garlic
2 tablespoons	dried onion flakes
1 teaspoon	coarse salt
½ teaspoon	pepper, freshly ground
½ teaspoon	paprika
1 cup	Arborio rice
1 cup	chicken stock (recipe on page 33)
2 cups	water (or you can use all broth or all water or ½ & ½, just so you have 3 cups of liquid)

Pressure cooker method: Heat the oil and butter in cooker over medium heat. Add the garlic, onions, salt, pepper, paprika and stir a few times. Stir in the rice and stir until opaque, about 1-2 minutes. Add unheated chicken stock, and or water. Lock the lid in place, bring to high pressure over high heat. Adjust the heat to maintain high pressure. Cook for 8 minutes. Release the pressure according to manufacturers instructions. Carefully open (be careful of the steam). Stir, cover and let sit for about 5 minutes until all the liquid is absorbed.

Stove top method: Melt the oil and butter in large saucepan. Add the garlic, onions, salt, pepper, and paprika and stir a few times. Stir in the rice and stir until opaque, about 1- 2 minutes. Heat the stock and or water in another pan. Stir 1 cup of hot liquid into the rice mixture stirring constantly until the rice absorbs almost all of the liquid, about 3 minutes. Add another cup and stir until almost absorbed. Repeat, keeping the risotto at a steady simmer and adding more liquid as needed until you use all the liquid and the rice is tender, about 20 minutes total. If you run out of liquid and the rice isn't tender, use hot water.

Note: For Spanish rice, just add salsa to cooked plain rice (Pace Chunky Salsa or recipe on page 73).

Note: You can add 2 cups of butternut squash or sweet potato (peel, seed and cube). Toss with a little oil and spread on cookie sheet. Sprinkle with salt and pepper. Bake in 400 degree oven for about 30 minutes until tender. If you are pressure cooking, just cut in small cubes and place on top of rice. Mix well when done.

Note: For variety you can also use red, yellow or green peppers or leeks. Use different herbs such as sage, parsley or basil.

VEGETABLE DISHES

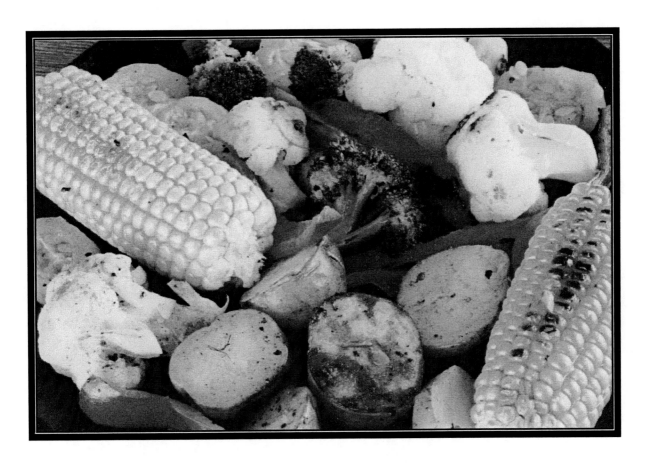

Grilled Vegetables, page 101

VEGETABLE STOCK

1 tablespoon	butter
1 tablespoon	canola or olive oil
½ cup	dried onion flakes
1 cup	carrots, chopped (approximately 2 carrots)
1 cup	parsnips, chopped (approximately 1 pound)
1 cup	celery, chopped, include some tops (approximately 2 stalks)
1 ½ pounds	Swiss chard
several	sprigs of fresh thyme
several	sprigs fresh parsley
2 dried	bay leaves

In a stockpot over medium heat melt butter and add oil. Add onion and stir until browned. Add carrots, parsnips, and celery. Cook for about 10 minutes. Wash and drain chard and chop. Add to other vegetables. Add 3 quarts of cold water, thyme, parsley and bay leaves. Bring to a boil, reduce heat and simmer for an hour. Remove from heat and strain stock through a strainer pressing on vegetables to extract juices. Discard vegetables. Refrigerate (use within 2 days or freeze).

SQUASH HASH

1 large	butternut squash, peeled, seeded, and cut into bite sized chunks
1 tablespoon	canola or olive oil
1 tablespoon	dried onion
2 teaspoons	garlic, minced
2 large	green chilies, de-seeded, roasted, peeled and chopped
1 large	red pepper, de-seeded, roasted, peeled and chopped
2 cobs	corn, kernals cut off
½ teaspoon	cumin
½ teaspoon	salt, coarse
1/4 teaspoon	pepper, freshly ground
2 tablespoons	cilantro, fresh, chopped

Bring water in a large pot to a boil. Prepare a bowl of ice water. Put chunks of squash (about 3-4 cups) into boiling water and cook for 3-4 minutes or until just barely tender. Drain in colander and place into ice water to stop cooking. Drain from ice water and spread on a cookie sheet to dry (if you want to do the day before, store in an airtight container in the refrigerator). Heat oil in large frying pan over medium heat. Add dry squash. Cook stirring occasionally for about 5 minutes. Add onion and garlic and stir. Cook and stir for another 5 minutes or so, until tender and browned. Add chilies, red pepper, corn, cumin, salt, pepper and cilantro. Stir until hot and well combined.

Serving Suggestion: This tastes great with grilled fish

ROASTED POTATO SPEARS

½ teaspoon	black pepper, freshly ground
½ teaspoon	thyme
½ teaspoon	garlic powder
½ teaspoon	lemon pepper
1 teaspoon	oregano
1 ½ teaspoons	salt
1/4 cup	melted butter
2 large	russet potatoes

Mix pepper, thyme, garlic powder, lemon pepper, oregano, and salt. Mix the butter and the herbs. Cut the potatoes lengthwise into 8 equal wedges. Toss the potatoes in the mixture. Place the potatoes on a cookie sheet lined with foil or Silpat and roast in a 400 degree oven for 20 minutes or until tender. Broil for a minute or two until browned, watch carefully so they don't burn.

POTATO RING

2 tablespoons	clarified butter (recipe on page 22) or 1 tablespoon of butter & 1 tablespoon oil
2 or 3 large	potatoes, un- peeled or peeled, and very thinly sliced (use a mandolin for best results)
	salt, coarse
	pepper, freshly ground

Heat 2 tablespoons of clarified butter (this is important because clarified butter does not burn as easily) in a 12" skillet (cast iron works best) over medium heat until very hot but not smoking. Working quickly, arrange potatoes in an overlapping circle, to fill bottom of pan, starting on outside with the biggest slices and working in using the smaller ones, making several layers (be careful because fat may splatter). Season each layer with salt and pepper. Brush the bottom of another pan (a little smaller than the other pan) with a little butter and place over the potatoes to weigh them down. Cook over medium heat until golden brown about 8 minutes. Flip the potatoes like a pancake, with a very large spatula, and cook the other side until brown, about another 8-10 minutes. Cut into wedges and serve immediately.

MASHED POTATOES

4-6	large russet potatoes, peeled and diced (1 potato per person) cut in ½ lengthwise, in ½ lengthwise again, put slices side by side and evenly dice
5	large garlic cloves, peeled (**optional**)
1 cup	milk
6 tablespoons	butter
1 ½ teaspoons	salt (or to taste)
1 teaspoon	freshly ground pepper (or to taste)

Cover potatoes and garlic with cold water in large pot. Put lid on pot and bring to a boil (about 20 minutes). Take lid off pot and cook until tender, approximately 15 minutes. While they cook, heat milk and butter over low heat (or microwave) until butter is melted and milk is warm. Drain cooked potatoes throughly and place in mixing bowl and whip with mixer for a minute or two and add butter, milk, salt and pepper and mix until as smooth as possible.

Note: Another way of making great mashed potatoes is to scrub the potatoes throughly with a vegetable brush, dice and cook with the skins on. The skins add a wonderful taste.

TWICE BAKED POTATOES

These potatoes are great to make for company as you can make them ahead of time., Cover and refrigerate for a couple of hours and bake 10-15 minutes before serving

4	large potatoes (nice fat potatoes, uniform in size) you'll have 8 halves
4 tablespoons	butter, melted
1 teaspoon	salt
½ teaspoon	pepper
1/8 teaspoon	paprika
1/8 teaspoon	white pepper
1/4 teaspoon	garlic powder
2 tablespoons	parsley
1 ½ cups	milk, warm
1 cup	natural cheddar cheese or farmers cheese, grated

Bake potatoes in a 400 degree oven for 1-1 ½ hours or until done (stick knife in center, should go through easily). Cut in half lengthwise and very carefully spoon out potato into large mixing bowl with slow lengthwise strokes leaving a bit on the bottom of the skin to keep it solid. Place skins on cookie sheet. Add to potatoes in mixing bowl: butter, salt, pepper, paprika, white pepper, garlic powder and parsley. Blend with mixer and add warm milk until right consistency and as smooth as possible. Spoon back into skins. Press grated cheese on top of each potato. Bake in a 400 degree oven for 10-15 minutes or until cheese is melted and potatoes are hot.

RED POTATOES AND VEGGIES

4 cups	red potatoes (approximately 20 small ones or 6 medium)
1 tablespoon	butter
1 cup	carrots, chopped
1	red pepper, chopped (roasted is best)
1	yellow pepper, chopped (roasted is best)
1	green pepper, chopped (roasted is best)

You may only need ½ of each pepper if they are very large, the 3 peppers diced should be about a cup

3/4 teaspoon	paprika
1 teaspoon	basil
½ teaspoon	thyme
1 teaspoon	salt
½ teaspoon	pepper
1 cup	farmer cheese, grated (optional) tastes great but if you want to keep the calories and fat down, leave it off

Steam potatoes until tender. Cool until you can handle and slice potatoes into ½" squares or cut small ones in half. Melt butter and mix with the potatoes and the rest of the ingredients, except for cheese, until well blended. Place in baking dish (if you want cheese, sprinkle on top) and bake in a 375 degree oven for 20 minutes.

Note: To save time, you can steam the potatoes the day before, wrap in foil and put in refrigerator.

POTATO PANCAKES (LATKES)

2	eggs
½ cup	dried onion flakes
1 teaspoon	salt
1/4 teaspoon	white pepper
1/4 teaspoon	garlic salt or garlic powder
1 teaspoon	baking powder
1 tablespoon	flour
1 pound (2 large)	potatoes (4 cups) unpeeled or peeled
	canola or olive oil
	creme fraiche (Vermont Butter and Cheese Co.) or sour cream (Daisy)
	applesauce (recipe on page 134 or "good" applesauce)

In a small bowl, whisk the eggs and add the onion, salt, pepper, garlic, baking powder, and flour. Shred potatoes into a large bowl. Immediately add the egg mixture and mix well until the potatoes are coated. (If you don't add the egg mixture right away, the potatoes will turn brown. You can cover them with water if you can't use them right away, but make sure you strain them well and pat dry with a paper towel before using). Pour olive oil to cover the bottom of a large skillet. Heat until very hot and add a large spoonful of potato mixture. Flatten a bit and turn when brown. Brown other side and drain on a brown paper bag (they stay crisper and don't stick the way they do on a paper towel). Serve hot with a dollup of creme fraiche or Daisy sour cream and applesauce.

SWEET POTATO CASSEROLE

6-8 cups	raw cubed sweet potatoes (approximately 3 large)
½ cup	milk
1/8 cup	sugar
3 tablespoons	butter
2	eggs
1 teaspoon	vanilla
½ teaspoon	salt

Cover cubed potatoes with water and boil until tender. Drain and place in mixing bowl. Mix on low speed until smooth. Add milk, sugar, butter, eggs, vanilla and salt. Pour into 2 quart baking dish.

Topping:

½ cup	brown sugar
1/4 cup	all purpose flour
1/4 cup	butter

Sprinkle over potato mixture and bake in a 350 degree oven for 35 minutes.

MASHED YAMS

2 medium	yams or sweet potatoes (4 cups diced raw)
2 tablespoons	butter
2 tablespoons	brown sugar
1/4 teaspoon	salt

Peel and cut yams into same size cubes. Cover with water and boil until tender. Drain well and put into mixing bowl. Add butter, sugar and salt. Beat with electric mixer until very smooth.

Serving Suggestion: tastes great with pork chops or pork roast

TONY AND FRAN'S CASSEROLE

2 teaspoons	garlic, minced
1 pound	asparagus tips, fresh
2 tablespoons	extra virgin olive oil
1 pound	peas, fresh or frozen
1 pound	artichoke hearts, fresh or "good" canned
5	eggs
1 teaspoon	pepper, freshly ground

Saute garlic and asparagus in oil for about a minute. Add peas and artichoke hearts until tender. Add eggs without breaking yolks. Sprinkle with pepper, cover and turn off heat. Let set for fifteen minutes and serve immediately.

BROCCOLI CASSEROLE

2 tablespoons	butter
2 tablespoons	flour
½ teaspoon	salt
1/4 teaspoon	white pepper
1 ½ cups	milk
½ cup	natural cheddar or farmer cheese, grated
2	eggs
3 cups	broccoli, washed, drained well and tops finely chopped
1/3 cup	finely crushed "good"corn flakes or crackers (optional)

Melt butter in saucepan on low heat, stir in flour, salt and pepper until smooth. Add milk gradually stirring constantly over medium heat until thickened and smooth. Add cheese and stir until well blended and melted.

Beat eggs in large bowl and add broccoli. Mix until well blended. Lightly spray an 8" x 8" baking pan and add broccoli mixture. Spoon on sauce. Sprinkle crumbs on top. Bake in a 325 degree oven, covered for 20 minutes, uncovered for 25 minutes or until set, toothpick inserted in center comes out clean.

STUFFED ZUCCHINI

1 medium	zucchini
1	tomato
1 teaspoon	butter
1	beaten egg
	salt and freshly ground pepper to taste
	grated farmer cheese

Cut the zucchini in half lengthwise. Scrape pulp into bowl leaving a little in shell. Place zucchini cut side down in frying pan with a little water. Bring to a boil, cover and simmer 5 minutes. Drain and turn right side up.

Finely chop pulp and tomato. Melt butter and saute pulp and tomato for about 2- 3 minutes. Add beaten egg, salt and pepper. Stirring constantly, cook until egg is well mixed and done. Spoon mixture into shells. Top with grated cheese and bake in a 350 degree oven until cheese melts.

ASPARAGUS

1 bunch	asparagus spears, thin, but not too thin, and firm

Asparagus is best eaten the day it is bought, but if you must refrigerate it, wrap the stem ends in damp paper towels, seal in an airtight plastic bag and leave it in the crisper for no more than three days. When you are ready to cook it, snap off the toughest end of the stems, they break naturally where the toughness stops. Peel the skin from the bottom third of any thick stalks and bind the bundle with kitchen string.

A good way to cook asparagus is to stand it on end in a few inches of water. Boil water in a small saucepan, add the asparagus and invert another saucepan over the top for a lid. Cook until the stalks are barely tender.

GLAZED CARROTS AND GREEN BEANS

Most of the sugar boils away when you cook this glaze. It adds just a little buttery sweetness to the vegetables

1 cup	water
1/4 cup	brown sugar
2 cups	carrots, peeled and sliced in bite sized pieces
2 cups	green beans, de-stringed, and broken in bite sized pieces
½ tablespoon	butter
1/4 teaspoon	salt

Bring water and brown sugar to a boil. Boil for about 10 minutes or until thickened and syrupy. While it is cooking prepare the carrots and beans.

Bring water in steamer to a boil. Add carrots and beans, cover and steam for about 5 minutes or until still crunchy but tender. Drain and place in bowl.

Add butter and salt to thickened sugar and water and stir well. Stir into vegetables.

HONEY GLAZED CARROTS

2 teaspoons	butter
1/4 cup	water
1/4 teaspoon	salt, coarse
3 cups	carrots, peeled and sliced into same size "sticks"
2 teaspoons	butter
1 tablespoon	honey

Heat 2 teaspoons of butter, water, and salt in a medium frying pan. Add the carrot sticks. Cover and cook on low heat for 5 minutes. Shake pan occasionally. Take off the cover, turn up the heat a little and stir and cook for about 5 more minutes or until most of the liquid is gone and the carrots brown a little. Add the remaining 2 teaspoons of butter and the honey. Stir and cook until carrots are glazed. Serve immediately.

STIR FRY CABBAGE

3 tablespoons	olive or canola oil
8 cups	cabbage, chopped
1 teaspoon	salt, coarse
½ teaspoon	pepper, freshly ground
1 tablespoon	sugar
2 tablespoons	dried onion flakes

Heat oil in wok or large frying pan. Add cabbage, salt, pepper, sugar and onions. Stir fry until cabbage is cooked and ingredients are well mixed. Doesn't take very long. Serve immediately.

99

EGGPLANT ZUCCHINI CASSEROLE

2 cups	tomatoes, fresh, diced (or 14 ounce can of diced tomatoes)
1 tablespoon	tomato paste
1 tablespoon	garlic, minced
½ teaspoon	sugar
2 tablespoons	basil, fresh, chopped (or 1 tablespoon dried)
1/4 teaspoon	salt, coarse
1/4 teaspoon	pepper, freshly ground
2 tablespoons	olive or canola oil
1 small	eggplant, peeled, sliced thin (but not too thin)
3 small	zucchini's (sliced thin, but not too thin)
4 ounces	mozzarella, fresh, sliced

Combine tomatoes, tomato paste, garlic, sugar, basil, salt and pepper in saucepan. Simmer on low heat for about 20-30 minutes. While sauce is simmering, prepare vegetables.

Heat oil in large frying pan. Place sliced eggplant in pan and saute until light brown on each side. Do the same with the zucchini. Place in oven proof baking dish. Pour sauce over the vegetables and lay the sliced cheese on top. Bake in a 350 degree oven for 15 minutes or until cheese is melted.

SQUASH CASSEROLE

6 cups (4 or 5)	zucchini or yellow squash or a combination of both, scrubbed and cut into 1/2" rounds
1/8 cup	onion flakes
1 teaspoon	coarse salt
1 teaspoon	freshly ground pepper
1 teaspoon	thyme, fresh or ½ teaspoon dried
1/8 teaspoon	cayenne
2	eggs, beaten together with milk
½ cup	milk (or if you want richer, use cream (Alta Dena)
1 cup	cheddar, natural white
½ cup	fine bread crumbs (optional)

In a large bowl, mix the squash, onion, salt, pepper, thyme, cayenne, beaten eggs and milk, and 1/4 cup of the cheese. Place in a 2 quart casserole dish. Spread remaining cheese and (optional) breadcrumbs on top. Cover and bake in a 350 degree oven until set, approximately 40 minutes. Turn up oven to 400 degrees, uncover and bake until top is browned, about 10 minutes.

SAUTEED VEGGIES

2 tablespoons	butter
2 teaspoons	garlic, minced
2	carrots, julienne sliced
1	zucchini, julienne sliced
1	red pepper, julienne sliced
1	yellow pepper, julienne sliced
1	green pepper, julienne sliced
1 small	jicama, julienne sliced
2 stalks	celery, julienne sliced
	coarse salt and freshly ground pepper

Melt butter in medium saucepan over low heat. Add garlic and stir a few times. Add the rest of veggies and stir fry quickly until crispy tender. Add salt and pepper to taste.

Note: Use any combination of veggies that you like

GRILLED VEGETABLES

3	zucchini (small, scrubbed and sliced)
1	yellow pepper, seeded, ends removed and sliced
2	stalks of peeled celery, diced
3 large	garlic cloves, skinned and cut in half
2-3 tablespoons	butter
	salt, pepper and paprika

Place sliced vegetables in heavy duty grill bag or on a heavy duty sheet of foil. Add garlic and butter and sprinkle with salt, pepper and paprika. Place another piece of foil on top and seal edges (or roll edges of grill bag). Grill, covered, on low heat, top shelf for about 20-25 minutes (depending on your particular grill). After about 10 to 15 minutes turn foil over or if in bag shake and turn over.

Note: Yellow squash is great cooked this way or any other vegetable combinations.

BAKED ARTICHOKE

Snap off tough outer bottom leaves. Cut off upper third of artichoke. Snip remaining leaf tips with scissors. Trim long stem leaving a flat bottom. Place ½ cup water in bottom of baking dish. Spray artichoke with a little olive oil. Cover. Bake in a 350 degree oven until heart is soft when pierced with the tip of a knife, about 30-40 minutes.

Pull off leaves and dip inner part of leaf into butter or mayonnaise and scrape off meat with teeth. Take out middle, heart, and with small knife scrape off hair. Slice and dip in butter or mayo.

Note: You can also stuff the artichoke by spreading the leaves away from center, revealing the choke. Remove choke with a spoon and discard. Mix bread crumbs, grated cheese, a little oil, parsley, oregano, salt and pepper. Spread the leaves and fill the artichoke and bake the same way as above, but take off the foil and bake for another 10 minutes for bread crumbs to brown.

SUNCHOKES (Jerusalem Artichokes)

I saw these interesting little potato looking things in the grocery store and was fascinated by them. I'm always looking for something new in the produce department so I decided to experiment with them. Through research I found that they are the roots of wild sunflowers. They are starch free and are a good source of iron and niacin. They are sweet and nutty tasting and are very versatile. You can keep sunchokes for up to 2 weeks in a plastic bag. Don't buy or use if they are soft. Scrub with a stiff vegetable brush under running water. You can steam, boil, bake or saute them. You can even dice raw and use in salad.

> olive oil & butter
> green, red or yellow peppers (or a combination of them)
> carrots
> sunchokes (Jerusalem artichokes)

Scrub sunchokes with a stiff vegetable brush under running water. Boil for 7 minutes. Cool and dice. Cut peppers in half and take out seeds. Dice. Scrub carrots, cut off ends and dice. Heat a little olive oil and butter in a small frying pan. Add diced vegetables and saute until vegetables are tender. Add salt and pepper to taste.

CORN RELISH

½ teaspoon	Spice Hunter Fish Seasoning (or a little thyme & parsley)
2	ripe tomatoes, cut in half and seeds squeezed out (throw away) and other part diced
1	red pepper, diced
16 ounces (2 cups)	frozen sweet white corn or fresh corn, cut off cob
½ teaspoon	salt
½ teaspoon	pepper
½ teaspoon	lemongrass ginger oil
1 tablespoon	butter
1 teaspoon	garlic, minced

In a bowl, mix together the fish seasoning, tomatoes, red pepper, corn, salt and pepper. Heat the oil and butter and stir in the garlic for a few seconds. Add the tomato mixture and stir until well blended and hot.

SAUTEED CORN MEDLEY

½ teaspoon	canola or olive oil
2 tablespoons	butter
1 teaspoon	garlic, minced
1 teaspoon	salt, coarse
½ teaspoon	pepper, freshly ground
1 cup	red pepper, diced
1 cup	celery, chopped
2 cups	corn, cut off the cob or frozen sweet white corn, thawed (thaw quickly by putting package in a bowl of cold water, rinse and drain throughly)

Heat oil and butter in small frying pan and add garlic, salt and pepper. Stir a few times and add red pepper and celery. Stir and saute over medium heat for 2 minutes. Turn heat up a little and add corn and stir and cook for two more minutes.

CREAMED CORN

Corn on the cob (how ever many you want), husked, de-silked

Using a corn cutter and creamer (can be bought at most kitchen stores) or a sharp knife, cut off corn, using a little pressure so you get the cream also.

Melt butter in frying pan over low heat and add corn, and salt and pepper to taste.

Cook just until tender, doesn't take very long. It is so good, it is really worth the effort!

SPAGHETTI SQUASH

6-7 pound	spaghetti squash
4 tablespoons	butter
4 tablespoons	parsley, fresh, chopped
	salt, coarse
	pepper, freshly ground

Cut squash in half lengthwise, spoon out and discard seeds. Place squash halves cut side down in a large pan. Add 2 cups of water, cover with foil. Bake in a 350 degree oven for about 50-60 minutes until squash is translucent and flesh pulls away from skin. Cool for 5 minutes. Using a fork, separate flesh into strands. Discard skins. Combine squash strands with butter, parsley, salt and pepper or with Spaghetti Sauce (recipe in Pasta section of book) or Fresh Tomato Sauce (recipe in Sauce section of book).

ROGER'S RED CABBAGE AND APPLES

3 cups	red cabbage, shredded
1 tablespoon	canola oil
1 large	apple, peeled, cored and sliced in bite sized pieces
1/8 cup	brown sugar
1 teaspoon	salt
1/4 cup	brown rice vinegar
1/4 cup	water

Heat oil in large frying pan. Add cabbage and saute for a minute. Add apples. Add brown sugar, salt, vinegar, and water. Simmer until most of the liquid is gone, about 3-5 minutes.

Serving Suggestion: This tastes great with roasted pork or pork chops

SAUTEED SWISS CHARD

1 ½ pounds	Swiss chard, washed
1 tablespoon	salt
1 tablespoon	olive or canola oil
1 tablespoon	dried onion
1-2 teaspoons	garlic, minced
1/4 teaspoon	cayenne pepper
1/4 teaspoon	salt, or to taste

In a large pot, bring 3 quarts of water to a boil. Cut off chard stems. When water reaches a boil, add 1 tablespoon salt. Add stems, cover and cook for 3 minutes. Add leaves, cover and cook for 3 more minutes. Drain in colander, rinse under cold water until cool. Drain again squeezing to remove any excess liquid. Chop. In a skillet heat oil over medium heat. Add onion and garlic. Stir until lightly browned. Stir in cayenne pepper and salt. Add chard, cayenne pepper and salt. Stir fry over medium heat until done.

SALADS

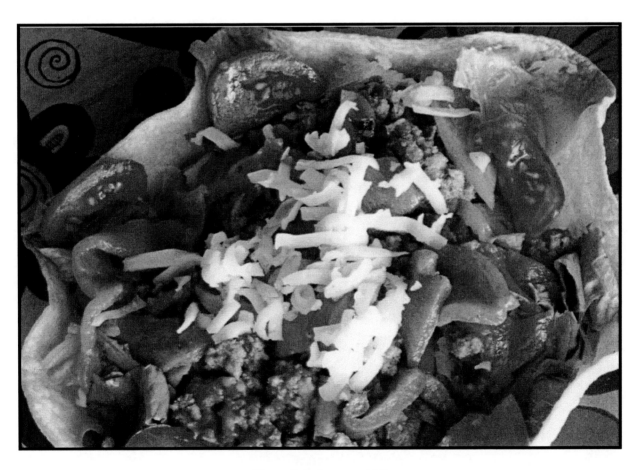

Taco Salad, page 112

SALAD TIPS

1. A variety of fresh lettuce and fresh herbs make a beautiful and delicious salad.

2. Always wash and sort lettuce, picking out only the good leaves. Wash in icy cold water, it helps to crisp it up.

3. Only use very fresh greens.

4. After washing and sorting, spin dry with salad spinner. Dressing will not stick to wet leaves.

5. Store lettuce in large zipper bag with a piece of paper towel (helps to keep moisture off of leaves)

GRILLED CHICKEN SALAD

chicken breasts sprinkled with Chicken Rub (recipe on page 33)
grilled, cooled and diced

romaine lettuce, outer leaves removed, inside crisp leaves chopped
tomato, diced
carrot, diced
broccoli, diced
cauliflower, diced
farmer cheese, grated

Mix together with dressing (recipes on pages 130 and 131)

CHICKEN SALAD

4	chicken breasts rubbed with Chicken Rub (recipe on page 33) grilled, cooled and diced
	mayonnaise (recipe on page 129)
4 stalks	celery, peeled and diced
1	red pepper, de-seeded, roasted peeled, and diced
	salt, coarse
	pepper, freshly ground

Combine, chicken, mayonnaise (to the consistency that you like), celery and red pepper. Add salt and pepper to taste.

Note: You can also make a really good chicken salad by boiling a whole chicken, pull apart and finely chop 4 cups of good breast meat. Add 1-1 ½ cups of mayonnaise and 1 cup of chopped celery, and 1-2 tablespoons of mustard (Rothschild or homemade, recipe in Sauce section of book), ½ teaspoon salt and ½ teaspoon pepper.

Serving Suggestion: Great on "good" french bread, Honey Oatmeal Bread, French Bread or Wheat Bread (recipes 120 and 121) with lettuce with tomato slices.

GRILLED CHICKEN PASTA SALAD

3-4	chicken breasts sprinkled with Chicken Rub (recipe on page 33) grilled, cooled, and diced
1	red pepper, de-seeded, roasted, peeled and chopped
½ cup	radishes (approximately 8), chopped
½ cup	jicama, chopped
½ cup	carrots, chopped
1 cup	celery, chopped
3-4	hardboiled eggs, chopped
8 ounces	small macaroni, cook according to package directions, drain in colander and rinse in cool water
2 cups	mayonnaise (recipe on page 129)
cup	creme fraiche (Vermont Butter and Cheese Co. or sour cream (Daisy)
1 tablespoon	mustard (recipe on page 129 or Rothschild Apricot Ginger)
1 teaspoon	horseradish (Bubbies)
½ teaspoon	Spice Hunter Caribbean Rub (or a little paprika, ginger, garlic, allspice, thyme)
1 tablespoon	rice vinegar
2 teaspoons	balsamic vinegar (Wild Thymes Cranberry Ginger)
2 teaspoons	salt, coarse
1 teaspoon	pepper, freshly ground

In a large bowl mix mayonnaise, creme fraiche or sour cream, mustard, horseradish, Caribbean Rub, rice vinegar, balsamic vinegar, salt, and pepper. Reserve ½ cup. Add the cooled, cooked macaroni, grilled chicken, red pepper, radishes, jicama, carrots, celery, and eggs to the bowl of dressing.

Cover and refrigerate for about an hour (dressing will absorb into macaroni). Mix in remaining ½ cup of dressing. Refrigerate until ready to serve.

Serving Suggestion: Great served with Honey Oatmeal Bread, Wheat Bread, Yeast Rolls (recipes on pages 120, 122, 127)

Note: If you like a lot of spice add a little cayenne, dry mustard or paprika to taste

OVERNIGHT LAYERED SALAD

6 cups	iceberg lettuce, chopped
2/3 cup	celery, chopped
1	red pepper, roasted and diced
1 cup	frozen peas
2/3 cup	jicama, chopped
1 cup	mayonnaise (recipe on page 129)
2-3	hardboiled eggs, sliced
1-2	tomatoes, sliced

Take off outer leaves of lettuce, use only the inner crisp leaves. Chop and place in a 9"x 9" casserole dish. Sprinkle celery, red pepper, peas, and jicama over lettuce. Spread mayonnaise evenly on top. Don't mix together. Put plastic wrap over and seal tightly. Serve next day, or make in the morning for dinner. Place the hardboiled eggs, and tomato slices on top.

OVERNIGHT MARINATED VEGGIE SALAD

This is an unusual salad that most people love. It is sweet and tangy. I double this recipe when I take it to a party

14 ounces	green beans, french style
16 ounces	peas, small, frozen
11 ounces	shoepeg corn (Green Giant)
	or frozen sweet white corn
3/4 cup	celery, chopped
1	red pepper, chopped (roasted tastes the best)
1/4 cup	canola or olive oil
3/4 cup	vinegar, white
½ cup	sugar
½ teaspoon	salt, coarse
½ teaspoon	pepper, freshly ground

Drain beans and combine with peas, corn, celery and pepper in a 9" x 13" pan. In saucepan heat oil, vinegar, sugar, salt and pepper until sugar is dissolved. Let cool and pour over veggies. Cover and refrigerate over night or make early in the morning. Stir occasionally. Put in serving bowl and serve with slotted spoon.

Note: Can add diced fresh tomatoes, finely diced cauliflower, broccoli, zucchini, fresh artichoke hearts, asparagus

CHOPPED SALAD

4 ears	corn, fresh, husked and hair removed
1/4 pound	green beans, trimmed and cut into 1/4" pieces
½ cup	peas, fresh (pop out of pods)
6	tomatoes, plum or roma, de-seeded and cut into 1/4" pieces
1 small	red pepper, de-seeded, deveined, and cut into 1/4" pieces
1 small	yellow pepper, de-seeded, deveined and cut into 1/4" pieces
1	cucumber, peeled, de-seeded, and cut into 1/4" pieces
1 cup	carrots, peeled and cut into 1/4" pieces
1 cup	celery, peeled and cut into 1/4" pieces
2 tablespoons	cilantro, fresh, chopped

Place cleaned corn into boiling water and boil for 6 minutes. Immediately put into a bowl of ice water. When corn is cool, remove, and using a large knife, remove kernels from corn. Place in large bowl. Add beans to boiling water and blanch for 1 minute. With a slotted spoon, remove and place in bowl of ice water. When cool, pour through a colander and place in bowl with corn. Add the rest of the vegetables and toss with Vinaigrette (recipe on page 131).

CHOPPED SALAD #2

large bunch	romaine, crisp inside leaves, washed, spun dry and chopped
2 large	carrots, peeled and chopped
1 cup	corn (fresh, cut off cob or thawed frozen)
1	jicama, peeled and chopped
2-3	tomatoes, chopped
1 cup	celery, peeled and chopped
1/4 cup	radishes, shredded

Combine and toss with dressing (recipes on pages 130 and 131)

ASPARAGUS AND JICAMA SALAD

romaine lettuce, outer leaves removed, crisp inside leaves chopped
hardboiled egg, diced
jicama, diced
tomato, diced
carrot, diced
asparagus, steamed and diced

Combine and toss with Vinaigrette (recipe on page 131)

SPINACH VEGGIE AND FRUIT SALAD

1 cup	spinach leaves, washed very well, spun dry and chopped
½ cup	carrots, peeled and diced
½ cup	jicama, peeled and diced
1	small apple, peeled, cored and diced
1/8 cup	dried cranberries (Sunsweet Cranberry Fruitlings)
1/4 cup	cherry tomatoes, cut in half

Mix all ingredients and serve with Creamy Salad Dressing (recipe on page 130).

CUCUMBER SALAD

4 cups	cucumbers, peeled and thinly sliced
1 cup	boiling water
½ cup	creme fraiche (Vermont Butter and Cheese Co.) or sour cream (Daisy)
1 teaspoon	sugar
1 tablespoon	raspberry vinegar (Wild Thymes)
1 tablespoon	dill, fresh (or 1 teaspoon dill seed)
1/4 teaspoon	salt
1/4 teaspoon	pepper

Pour boiling water over peeled and sliced cucumbers. Drain immediately in colander, place in bowl and cover with ice water. Drain again and dry (lay on towel, another one on top and blot). Mix creme fraiche or sour cream, sugar, vinegar, dill, salt and pepper. Toss with cucumbers and refrigerate.

Serving Suggestion: This salad tastes great with salmon cakes or any other fish recipe

COLE SLAW

4 cups	cabbage, shredded (can use ½ green and ½ red cabbage)
1 cup	carrots, chopped
½ cup	mayonnaise (recipe on page 129)
½ cup	creme fraiche (Vermont Butter and Cheese Co.)or sour cream (Daisy)
1 tablespoon	mustard (recipe on page 129 or Rothschild)
1 tablespoon	vinegar, apple cider
1 tablespoon	sugar
½ teaspoon	salt
1	apple, diced
½ cup	dried cranberries or cherries (Cranberry Fruitlings or Mariani Cherries)

Take off outer leaves of cabbage and shred or chop the rest making 4 cups. Chop the carrots. Mix the mayonnaise, creme fraiche or sour cream, mustard, vinegar, sugar and salt. Stir into cabbage mixture. Add apples and cranberries and mix well. Refrigerate until ready to serve.

EGG WHITE SALAD

I like to cut down on fat whenever I can and this salad tastes as good as egg salad using the yolks. Egg whites have 3.5 grams of protein, 0 fat, 0 carbs. Hardboiled eggs are 70% fat, 6.9 grams, 6.2 grams protein, 0 carbs.

6	hardboiled eggs (recipe on page 22) peeled, yolks removed and whites chopped
4-6 tablespoons	mayonnaise (recipe on page 129)
1 teaspoon	mustard, (recipe on page 129 or Rothschild)
1/3 cup	celery, peeled and diced
1/4 - ½ teaspoon	salt, coarse (to taste)
1/4 - ½ teaspoon	pepper, freshly ground (to taste)
	romaine (crisp inner leaves), washed and spun dry

Serving Suggestion: Place romaine leaves in bowl. Mix ingredients together and place on leaves. Also very good on Oatmeal Honey Bread or Wheat Bread (recipes on pages 120 and 121)

TUNA SALAD

2 - 6 ounce cans	"good" tuna
	mayonnaise (recipe on page 129)
	mustard (recipe on page 129 or Rothschild)
2 stalks	celery, peeled and diced
2	hardboiled eggs, diced
2	tomatoes, fresh, diced
	salt and pepper to taste

Drain tuna and stir in mayonnaise and mustard (to taste) until creamy. Add the celery, eggs, tomatoes, salt and pepper. Serve on crisp romaine leaves or on "good" bread.

POTATO SALAD

3	potatoes
2 cups	mayonnaise (recipe on page 129, double recipe)
2 tablespoons	mustard (recipe on page 129 or Rothschild Raspberry Honey)
1 cup	celery, diced
3	hardboiled eggs, diced

Place whole potatoes in large pot, cover with water and bring to a boil. Turn down heat and simmer until done (stick knife in center of largest potato to see if it is soft). Take out and place in large bowl to cool in refrigerator. When cool, peel and dice (should be about 5 cups). Mix mayonnaise and mustard to taste. Mix with diced potatoes. Add celery and eggs and refrigerate

TACO SALAD

1 pound	ground sirloin or lean ground beef
1/4 cup	dried onion flakes
1 teaspoon	garlic, minced
1 teaspoon	salt
1 teaspoon	chile powder
1 teaspoon	cumin
14 ounces	diced tomatoes (Eden Organic)
1	red pepper, de-seeded, roasted, peeled, and sliced
1	yellow pepper, de-seeded, roasted, peeled, and sliced
2 or 3	green chiles, de-seeded, roasted, peeled, and sliced
2 cups	romaine lettuce (outer leaves removed, use crisp inner leaves) diced
2 or 3	tomatoes, fresh, diced
½ cup	white cheddar or farmer cheese, grated
½ cup	Creamy Dressing (recipe on page 130)

Saute beef until brown. Drain off liquid and add onion, garlic, salt, chile powder, and cumin. Stir in tomatoes and simmer for 20 minutes. Add peppers and chiles and cool in refrigerator.

In a large bowl, mix cooled meat mixture, lettuce, tomatoes, cheese and dressing. Place equal amounts of mixture in each tortilla bowl (recipe below) or, you can heat tortillas in frying pan, sprinkle grated cheese on top until cheese is melted and tortilla is crisp. Slice with pizza cutter and put slices around the edge of each individual large bowl.

Tortilla Bowls:

Butter one side of each tortilla and form over an upside down oven proof bowl. Place upside down bowls on cookie sheet and bake in a 350 degree oven for 10 minutes until crispy. Take tortilla off of bowl and place right side up and let cool on plates.

Note: You can also use this filling for taco's. Just heat about ½ cup oil in a 9" small frying pan. When the oil is really hot, put a corn tortilla in pan. After just a second or two, fold over half of the tortilla with tongs. When good and crisp, turn over. Take out and place on paper towels to drain. Fill with meat mixture, and top with lettuce, tomatoes and cheese.

FRUIT SALAD

2 cups	peach slices, fresh, or canned
2 cups	apples, peeled, cored and sliced
2 cups	cherries, pitted, or canned
2 cups	blueberries, fresh, frozen or canned
2 cups	blackberries, fresh, frozen or canned
2 cups	watermelon, seeds removed and sliced into bite sized pieces
2 cups	pears, peeled, cored and sliced into bite sized pieces
2 cups	strawberries, fresh, sliced
	granola, recipe on page 157

Mix fruit together and just before serving, sprinkle a little granola on top of each serving.

If you want to mix the fruit with a sweet dressing, try the recipes below.

1 cup (8 ounces)	cream cheese, softened (Gina Marie)
2 tablespoons	fruit juice
1 cup (8 ounces)	heavy whipping cream (Alta Dena)
1/4 cup	sugar
½ teaspoon	pure vanilla

Mix softened cream cheese with fruit juice until well blended and set aside. Whip cream with sugar and vanilla until stiff peaks form. Stir cream cheese mixture and whipped cream together until well blended.

Or:

½ cup	cream cheese (Gina Marie)
1/4 cup	butter
1 cup	powdered sugar
½ teaspoon	vanilla
1 cup	creme fraiche (Vermont Butter and Cheese Co. or Daisy sour cream)

Or: creme fraiche plain or mixed with a little honey, cinnamon and nutmeg.

Or: mix fruit with whipped cream

Serving Suggestion: layer fruit and dressing in a glass bowl, and refrigerate until serving.

TABOULI SALAD
(Middle Eastern Wheat Salad)

I discovered tabouli at an Herb Association meeting I recently attended. The main ingredient is bulgur wheat. I had never heard of bulgur wheat and decided to research it a bit. This is what I found out: bulgur is a quick cooking form of whole wheat that has been cleaned, parboiled, dried, ground into particles and sifted into distinct sizes. The result is a nutritious, low fat, versatile wheat product with a pleasant, nut-like flavor and an extended shelf-life that allows it to be stored for long periods. It is similar to rice or couscous but has a higher nutritional value. It is ready to eat with minimal cooking or, after soaking in water or broth, can be mixed with other ingredients without further cooking. Use it as a side dish mixed with seasonings, vegetables, etc. instead of rice or use it in soup, stuffing, or casseroles.

½ cup	bulgur wheat
1 cup	boiling water
3 or 4	tomatoes, fresh, de-seeded and finely chopped
1 cup (1 large)	cucumber, fresh, peeled, de-seeded and finely chopped
1 or 2 teaspoons	garlic, minced
2 tablespoons	mint, fresh, chopped
1 cup	parsley leaves, fresh, packed and then chopped
1/4 cup	cranberry ginger balsamic vinegar (Wild Thymes) (traditionally lemon juice is used, but since citrus can be a trigger, I used vinegar instead)
1/4 cup	olive oil
½ teaspoon	salt, coarse
1/4 teaspoon	pepper, freshly ground

Soak bulgur wheat in boiling water for ½ an hour. Cut tomatoes in half and gently squeeze out seeds. Discard seeds and finely chop the rest. Peel cucumber, cut cucumber in half lengthwise, scrape out seeds with spoon and discard and finely chop the rest. In a medium bowl, combine the bulgur, tomatoes, cucumber, garlic, mint, and parsley together. In a container with a tight fitting lid, mix the vinegar, oil, salt and pepper together. Shake until well blended. Stir into the rest of the ingredients.

Serving Suggestion: Great on crackers, recipe on page 125 or "good" crackers (use a slotted spoon to drain off most of the liquid before putting on crackers)

114

SOUP

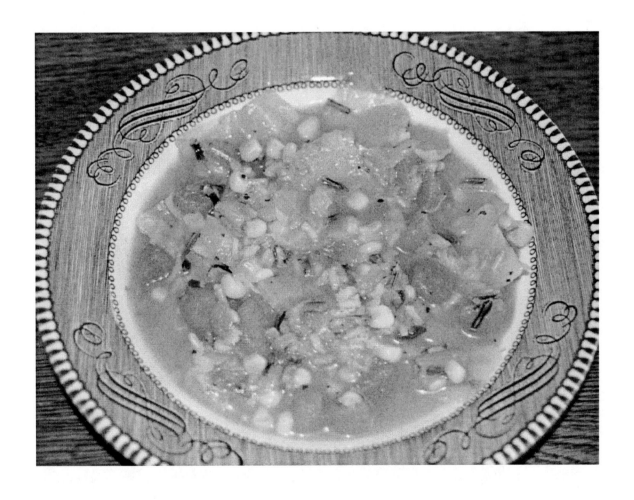

Chicken Soup, page 115

CHICKEN SOUP
I always make this soup when my family is sick, it really helps!

2   whole chickens, giblets removed and insides washed well

In very large pot place chickens and add water to cover. Bring to a boil and cook on medium heat (just so the water is bubbling) for 1-1 ½ hours or until done. Turn once or twice. Place on platter, pull apart with fork and let cool. When cool enough to handle, pull off good meat and discard skin and bones, etc. If you have time, cool broth and skim off fat from the top. A quick way is to add ice cubes (fat will cling to them and spoon off) or pour into fat separator. Add salt and pepper to taste. I always cook two chickens and freeze some of the broth and chicken for another meal.
Put the meat and broth you will need back into the pot.
Add the seasonings, to taste, that you like: basil, poultry seasoning, coriander, garlic powder, marjoram, parsley or sage. You can try a little of any of these seasonings in a little broth to see if that is what tastes good to you, or even a combination of several.
Add chopped carrots, celery, corn, beans, cabbage, dried onions, whatever vegetables you like. Add either noodles, rice, diced potatoes, dumplings or pierogi and simmer until vegetables are done (don't over-cook, you want the vegetables to be a little crunchy and the pasta "al dente")

Serving Suggestion: Hot buttered bread or rolls is perfect with this soup

VEGETABLE BEEF SOUP

1 tablespoon	canola oil
2 pounds	extra lean beef cubes cut in bite sized pieces
2 tablespoons	dried onion
1 teaspoon	garlic, minced
½ teaspoon	marjoram
1 teaspoon	salt
½ teaspoon	pepper
2 cups	water
4 cups	crushed tomatoes
3 cups	cubed potatoes (about 3 potatoes)
2 cups	carrots, thick slices
2 cups	celery
4 cobs	corn, kernals cut off
1-2 cups	cabbage, bite sized chunks

Heat oil in large kettle. Add beef and saute until brown. Add onions and garlic and cook and stir for a minute or two. Add marjoram, salt, and pepper. Stir water into meat. Add more water if needed to cover meat. Cook on low boil for an hour. Add tomatoes and simmer for 15 minutes. Taste and add more seasonings if needed. If you want more zest, add a little cayenne or paprika. Add potatoes and simmer for 10 minutes. Add carrots and cook for 10 more minutes. Add celery and corn. Cook until all vegetables are tender, about 10 more minutes. The last 5 minutes add the cabbage, cover pot and cook until tender.

Note: You can also add green beans or any other vegetable that you like. Don't overcook vegetables. This recipe makes a lot of soup. To avoid over-cooking vegetables, only re-heat the amount you know you will eat.

CORN CHOWDER

2	chicken breasts, rubbed with Chicken Rub on both sides (recipe on page 33) grilled and diced
3 tablespoons	butter
1 tablespoon	basil, fresh (or ½ tablespoon dried)
1/3 cup	dried onion flakes
1 cup	celery, finely chopped
2 teaspoons	salt
1 teaspoon	pepper, freshly ground
1	red pepper, de-seeded, roasted, peeled and finely diced
4 cups	corn, fresh (approximately 8 ears of corn) or frozen corn
4 cups	chicken stock (recipe on page 33)
1-2	potatoes (peeled or not peeled) finely diced
1 cup	milk (if you like richer you can use half and half or cream)

Cut corn off cob and set aside. Melt butter in small frying pan. Add basil, onion, celery, salt and pepper. Add red pepper and corn and stir. Add chicken stock and potatoes. Simmer until potatoes are done, approximately 30 minutes. Add milk and grilled chicken and stir for a minute or two until hot (don't bring to a boil once you have added the milk)

CLAM CHOWDER

2 tablespoons	butter
2 tablespoons	flour
1/4 cup	dried onion flakes
1 teaspoon	salt, coarse
½ teaspoon	pepper, freshly ground
1/8 teaspoon	paprika
1/8 teaspoon	white pepper
3 cups	milk
3 cups	diced red potatoes (peeled or unpeeled) steamed until tender
10 ounces	boiled baby clams (Crown Prince)

Melt butter and stir in flour. Add onion and cook for a minute or two. Add salt, pepper, paprika, white pepper and milk. Add cooked diced red potatoes and clams. Simmer on low, stirring occasionally, until hot (about 10 minutes).

SAUSAGE AND KALE SOUP

½ pound	sausage (recipe on page 61, Hans or Golden Farms Mild Italian)
1 tablespoon	dried onion flakes
1 teaspoon	garlic, minced
1 large	potato, peeled and cubed
5 cups	chicken stock (recipe on page 33)
3/4 teaspoon	pepper, freshly ground
1/8 teaspoon	paprika
	salt to taste
1 cup	kale leaves, washed and finely chopped

Saute sausage in small frying pan until done, add onion and garlic. Stir a few times and add potato. Stir a few more times. Drain off any excess oil being careful not to pour off any of the ingredients (pour through a fine strainer over sink). Add stock, pepper, paprika and salt to taste. Add chopped kale and simmer for a few minutes.

GREEN CHILI SOUP

1 tablespoon	olive or canola oil
1/4 cup	dried onion flakes
2 teaspoons	garlic, minced
1/8 cup	cilantro, fresh (or 1 tablespoon dried)
½ teaspoon	cumin
½ teaspoon	oregano, fresh (or 1/4 teaspoon dried)
3/4 tablespoon	salt, coarse
1/4 teaspoon	pepper, freshly ground
6 cups	chicken stock (recipe on page 33)
1	potato (peeled or not peeled) finely diced
1	carrot, finely diced
6	green chilies, de-seeded, roasted, peeled and finely diced
	"good" tortilla chips
	farmer cheese, grated

Heat oil in small frying pan and add onion, garlic, cilantro, cumin, oregano, salt and pepper. Saute for a minute or two until onion is soft but not brown. Pour broth in large pot and add sauteed ingredients, diced potatoes and carrots. Bring to a boil and simmer for 15 minutes and add diced chilies, simmer for 5 more minutes or until potatoes and carrots are tender.

To serve: put broken tortilla chips in the bottom of bowl. Spoon hot soup over chips and sprinkle grated cheese on top.

TOMATO SOUP

20	roma tomatoes, cored and halved lengthwise
	olive or canola oil
2 tablespoons	basil, fresh, chopped (or 1 tablespoon dried)
1 tablespoon	tarragon, fresh, chopped (or ½ tablespoon dried)
1 tablespoon	parsley, fresh, chopped (or ½ tablespoon dried)
3 cups	chicken stock (recipe on page 33)
½ teaspoon	coriander
½ teaspoon	cumin
1½ teaspoons	salt, coarse
½ teaspoon	pepper, freshly ground
1 tablespoon	cilantro, fresh, chopped (or ½ tablespoon dried)

Place the halved tomatoes cut side down on a large greased 12" x 17"cookie sheet or jelly roll pan. Cut an X on the skin side to score them. Brush or spray tomatoes with oil and sprinkle with the basil, tarragon and parsley. Roast in a 250 degree oven for two hours. Remove the tomatoes from the oven and puree in a blender or food processor until smooth. Place the puree in a saucepan and add the chicken stock. Season soup with the coriander, cumin, salt and pepper. Adjust amounts of seasonings to your liking. Bring to a boil. Reduce heat and simmer for ten minutes.

PUMPKIN SOUP

6 cups	chicken stock (recipe on page 33)
2-3 cups	sugar pumpkin, fresh, peeled, seeded, scrape off the strings and cut into ½" cubes
4 tablespoons	dried onion flakes
1 teaspoon	garlic, minced
1 ½ teaspoons	salt, coarse
1 teaspoon	thyme, fresh (or ½ teaspoon dried)
½ teaspoon	pepper, freshly ground
½ cup	heavy cream, warmed (do not boil)

In a medium saucepan heat the stock, pumpkin, onion, garlic, salt, thyme, and pepper. Cover and bring to a boil, reduce heat to low boil and simmer for 20 minutes. Puree mixture in a blender or food processor until smooth. Return to pot. Bring mixture to a boil, reduce heat and simmer uncovered for 10 minutes. Turn off heat and stir in the warm cream (after adding cream, do not boil soup).

SPICY SQUASH SOUP

2 tablespoons	olive oil
4 tablespoons	dried onion flakes
1 cup	celery, chopped
2 teaspoons	garlic, minced
2 teaspoons	curry, Madras style
1 ½ pounds (4 cups)	butternut squash, peeled, seeded and cubed
1 cup	green plantains, peeled and cut up (or 1 green banana)
6 cups	chicken broth (recipe on page 33)
½ teaspoon	dried oregano (or 1 teaspoon fresh
1 teaspoon	sage, fresh (or ½ teaspoon dried)
1/4 teaspoon	tabasco sauce
1 teaspoon	salt
½ teaspoon	pepper, freshly ground

Heat the oil in a Dutch oven, add onion and celery and saute for a minute. Add the garlic and stir a few times. Stir in the curry. Add the squash, plantains and broth. Add the oregano, sage, tabasco, salt and pepper. Bring to a boil, reduce heat and simmer on low boil, partially covered, for about 20 minutes or until squash is tender. Remove from heat and add, in batches, to blender or food processor and puree. Return to the pot and reheat. Garnish with croutons (recipe in Bread section of book) fresh chopped parsley or cilantro or grated cheese.

SPLIT PEA SOUP

I used to make this soup with a ham bone, but because ham is a "trigger", I made this recipe without the ham, and to my surprise, it tastes great!

2 teaspoons	canola or olive oil
1/4 cup	dried onion flakes
1 cup	carrots, peeled and diced
1 cup	celery, peeled and diced
2 ½ cups	chicken stock (recipe on page 33)
6 cups	water
1 cup	dried split peas
2 teaspoons	salt
1/8 teaspoon	thyme
1/8 teaspoon	marjoram
1 or 1 ½ teaspoons	salt, coarse (to taste)
½ teaspoon	pepper, freshly ground

In a medium saucepan, heat the oil and saute the onions until slightly brown. Add the carrots and celery and stir a few times. Add the chicken stock and stir to combine.

In a large pot, combine the water and peas. Bring to a boil and add salt. Simmer on low boil for about an hour. Add the vegetables and stock, thyme, marjoram, salt, and pepper. Continue simmering for another 30 minutes or until peas are tender.

POTATO AND LEEK SOUP

Leeks are a great alternative to onions and they add lots of flavor to this soup

1 ½ cups	leeks (2) thinly sliced and chopped (remove root end and tough green leaves from the top and one or two layers of the rest leaving only the tender part of the leek, rinse and drain well)
1 cup	celery, peeled and finely chopped
1 tablespoon	butter
4 cups	potatoes, peeled or unpeeled and diced (approximately 2 to 4 depending on size)
4 cups	water (or just enough to cover potatoes)
2 cups	milk
1/8 teaspoon	paprika
2-3 teaspoons	salt, coarse (to taste)
½ teaspoon	pepper, freshly ground

Melt butter in a large pot and add chopped leeks and celery. Stir and saute until cooked through, about a minute or two. Add diced potatoes and stir. Add water just to cover. Bring to a boil and simmer for about 15 minutes until potatoes are almost done. Add milk, paprika, salt and pepper. Simmer until potatoes are soft. Adjust seasonings if needed. If you want a thicker soup, add 2 tablespoons of flour to ½ cup of milk. Stir until smooth. Add to soup, stir constantly until thickened.

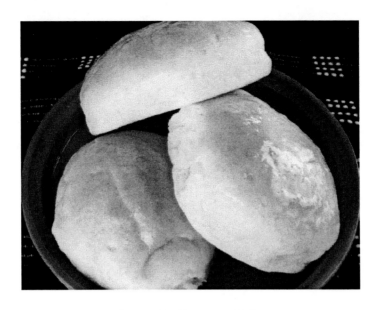

Yeast Rolls, page 122

BREADS, ROLLS, BISCUITS, MUFFINS, PANCAKES, CRACKERS, CROUTONS

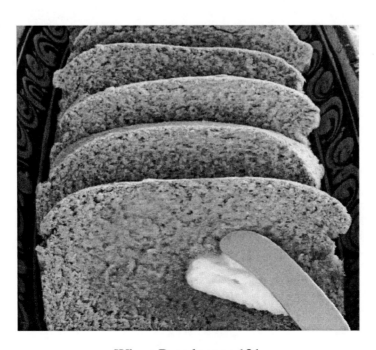

Wheat Bread, page 121

HONEY OATMEAL BREAD

Bread Maker Method:

1 cup	water
1 tablespoon	canola oil
1/4 cup	honey
1 teaspoon	salt
1 cup	oatmeal
2 cups	bread flour
2 ½ teaspoons	yeast (one package)

Add water, oil and honey to bread container. Add salt, oatmeal, bread flour and yeast. Start bread machine. Makes large **delicious** loaf.

Oven Method:

Place yeast in ½ cup of the water (warm) in a small bowl. Stir until dissolved. In a separate bowl, mix the other ½ cup of water with the oil and honey. In another bowl, mix the salt, oatmeal and flour together. Combine everything together until well blended. Knead on a lightly floured bread board for about 7 minutes. Shape into a ball and place a large inverted bowl over dough and let rise in a warm place for 60 minutes. Punch down and knead 10 times. Place bowl over dough and let rise for another 60 minutes. Punch down and knead 10 times and let rise for a final 60 minutes. Place in an oiled bread pan (gently shape to pan). Bake for 35-40 minutes until top is browned. Let cool for about 10 minutes before slicing.

FRENCH BREAD

3 ½ cups	bread flour
1 ½ teaspoons	sugar
1 1/4 teaspoons	salt
3 tablespoons	warm water (not hot)
1/4 ounce package	rapid rise yeast (or regular)
1 tablespoon	butter, melted (warm, not hot)
1 cup	water

In a large bowl, mix bread, sugar and salt. In a cup mix 3 tablespoons warm water with yeast and stir until smooth. Add warm butter and stir. Add to flour mixture along with 1 cup of water. Stir and form into a ball with your hands. Place on lightly floured surface and knead for 5 minutes until smooth and not sticky.

Place ball of dough in bowl and cover tightly with plastic wrap. Put in warm place and let rise until doubled about 1 to 1 ½ hours. Roll dough out into a 15"x 12" rectangle. Roll up tightly from long side, seal and taper ends. Place seam side down on greased baking sheet (or silpat lined). Cover with plastic wrap and let rise in warm, draft free place for 1 to 1 ½ hours or until nearly doubled in size. With a sharp knife make 4 quarter inch deep diagonal cuts on top of loaf. Bake in a 350 degree oven for 40 minutes. Cool slightly before slicing.

WHEAT BREAD

1 cup	water
2 tablespoons	honey
2 tablespoons	butter, softened
5 tablespoons	warm water (not hot)
1 ½ teaspoons	fast rise yeast
3 ½ cups	whole wheat flour (even better with freshly ground whole wheat)
1 ½ teaspoons	salt

In a small bowl, mix 1 cup of water with honey, and butter. In a small bowl or cup, mix 5 tablespoons of warm water with the yeast until well blended. In a large bowl, combine flour and salt and add the rest of ingredients. Form into a ball and knead for 5 minutes until smooth and not sticky. Place ball of dough in large bowl and cover tightly with plastic wrap. Put in a warm place and let rise until doubled in size, about 1 ½ hours. Punch down, knead a couple of times and repeat above. Let rise another hour. Punch down, knead a few times and let rise for another hour. Carefully place in large, lightly oiled bread pan. Bake in a 350 degree oven for 30-40 minutes or until done.

CINNAMON BREAD

1/3 cup	milk
2 tablespoons	butter
1 large	egg
1/4 cup	warm, not hot, water
1 package	yeast, regular or fast
1/8 teaspoon	sugar
2 1/4 cups	bread flour or unbleached all purpose flour
1 tablespoon	sugar
½ teaspoon	salt
1 teaspoon	cinnamon
2 tablespoons	sugar
2 tablespoons	butter, melted

Heat milk and butter in a small saucepan over low heat until milk is warm and butter is melted. In a small bowl, whisk the egg and add to the milk mixture. In another small bowl combine water, yeast and sugar. Stir until smooth. Sift the flour, sugar and salt into a mixer bowl. Using an electric mixer with a dough hook, gradually add the milk mixture until well combined. Add the yeast mixture and mix well. Scrape the sides when necessary. Place dough on clean work surface and knead for about 2 to 3 minutes until it is smooth and when pressed with your finger, the dough springs back. Place dough ball in a buttered bowl and cover tightly with plastic wrap. Put in a warm place and let rise until doubled. It takes about an hour. Combine the cinnamon and sugar. Place the dough on work surface, punch down and knead for about a minute. Roll out to a 8" x 12" rectangle. Spread on the melted butter and sprinkle the cinnamon sugar on top. Roll the 8" side of the dough, tucking and rolling tightly. Pinch the dough together when you reach the end to seal and also do the sides. Carefully place the dough, seam side down in a buttered 8" x 4" loaf pan. Cover with plastic wrap and put in warm place to rise. When dough has doubled in size and is at the top of the pan, about 30 minutes to an hour, place in a 350 degree oven for about 30-35 minutes or until golden brown. Brush the top with butter while it is still hot.

YEAST ROLLS

1 cup	hot water
1/4 cup	butter
2 tablespoons	sugar
1 teaspoon	salt
1/4 cup	warm, not hot, water
1 package	active dry yeast (25 ounce) regular not fast rising
3 cups	bread flour or unbleached all purpose flour
1	egg, slightly beaten

Place hot water in large bowl. Stir in cut up butter until it melts. Add sugar and salt. In a small bowl, add warm water and yeast and stir to dissolve yeast. Add to butter mixture. Add 1 ½ cups of flour and mix. Add egg. Add the rest of the flour and mix well. On a lightly floured surface with floured hands, knead a few times and work in just enough flour so the dough doesn't stick to your hands (be careful not to add too much flour, as the rolls won't be as tender). Form into a ball and place a large bowl and cover with plastic wrap. In a warm place, let rise until doubled (about an hour). Punch down, knead once and let rise 30 more minutes, covered, or until doubled in size.* Make egg sized balls of dough (12) and place about 2 inches apart on buttered baking sheet. Lightly cover with plastic wrap and let rise for 30 more minutes in a warm place. Bake in a 350 degree oven for 30 minutes or until lightly browned on top. Brush tops of rolls with butter while hot.

Note: *can leave the dough, covered, for a while if you don't want to bake right away. You can also place dough in a **large** zipper plastic bag (it will rise in the refrigerator) and refrigerate for the next day. Only keep one day though.

Note: You can also make cinnamon rolls out of this dough. After dough doubles in size, place on floured cutting board and roll out into a rectangle. Spread on melted butter and sprinkle with cinnamon sugar. Roll up (long end) and cut. Place on buttered cookie sheet, place in warm place and let rise until doubled. Bake in a 350 degree oven until browned, about 30 minutes.

BISCUITS

2 cups	unbleached all purpose flour
1 tablespoon	baking powder
3/4 teaspoon	salt
½ teaspoon	baking soda
5 tablespoons	butter, cold
1 cup	milk

In a large bowl sift together flour, baking powder, salt and baking soda. Cut the butter into small pieces and using a pastry blender or two knives, cut the butter into the flour mixture until coarse crumbs form. Add the milk, stir with fork until dough forms. Turn dough onto a lightly floured surface and form into a smooth, flat round 3/4" thick. Don't over handle the dough or the biscuits will be tough (the dough can be refrigerated up to 2 hours ahead, wrapped in plastic wrap). Using a biscuit cutter or a glass dipped in flour cut out biscuits. Place 2" apart on an ungreased baking sheet. Bake in a 450 degree oven for 12-15 minutes or until brown. Makes about 10.

Note: To make in a black iron dutch oven, preheat dutch oven for 15 minutes in a 450 degree oven. Spray lightly with oil and place biscuits in a circle, touching. Spoon a little melted butter on top. Cover and bake for 15 minutes. Take top off and broil until top is brown. These are great when you go camping. Put the dutch oven in the coals of a campfire and coals on top of the lid. Check after 10 minutes.

122

CORN MUFFINS

These muffins are wonderful! Not exactly low calorie but a nice treat once in a while. It's really worth the extra trouble of using fresh corn.

2 sticks	butter, softened
1 cup	sugar
½ cup	yellow cornmeal
½ cup	blue cornmeal (or can use 1 cup yellow cornmeal)
4	eggs
1 ½ cup	unbleached all purpose flour
1 tablespoon	baking powder
1 tablespoon	salt
1/3 cup	farmer cheese or white cheddar cheese, grated
1 3/4 cup	fresh corn (cut off the cob, make sure you cut deep to get the milk) or you can use a 14 ounce can of "good" creamed corn)

Cream butter, sugar and corn meal with a mixer until well blended. Add eggs one at a time beating until well blended after each. Add flour, baking powder and salt. Blend in cheese and corn. Evenly distribute batter into 12 large size, lightly oiled, muffin cups. Bake for 25-35 minutes in a 325 degree oven or until toothpick inserted in center comes out clean.

A smaller, little bit different version of this recipe is as follows:

1 stick	butter, softened
½ cup	sugar
½ cup	yellow cornmeal
2	eggs
1 cup	frozen corn
3/4 cup	unbleached, all purpose flour
½ tablespoon	baking powder
½ tablespoon	salt
1/4 cup	farmer cheese or white cheddar cheese

Same instructions as above. Makes 6 large muffins or 12 small ones.

CORNMEAL MUFFINS

1 1/4 cups	cornmeal
1 cup	unbleached all purpose flour
1/3 cup	packed brown sugar
1/3 cup	sugar
1 teaspoon	baking soda
½ teaspoon	salt
1	egg
1 cup	milk
3/4 cup	canola oil

In a bowl, combine cornmeal, flour, brown sugar, sugar, baking soda and salt. In another bowl, beat egg, milk and oil. Stir in dry ingredients just until moistened. Fill twelve oiled or paper-lined muffin cups three quarters full. Bake in a 425 degree oven for 12-15 minutes or until muffins test done (toothpick inserted in center should come out clean). Cool in pan for ten minutes before removing.

MEXICAN CORNBREAD

2 cups	creamed corn (cut off cob, cut deep into cob so you get some of the cream along with the kernals) or use frozen corn
4	green chiles, de-seeded, roasted, peeled, and diced (or 4 ounce can of "good" diced green chilies)
1	egg
1/3 cup	milk
1 cup	white cheddar cheese or farmer cheese, grated
1 cup	corn meal (Arrowhead Mills Yellow Cornmeal)
½ cup	bread flour
½ teaspoon	soda
1 teaspoon	salt
½ teaspoon	baking powder

Mix corn, green chilies, egg, and milk together. Add the cheese. Blend in the corn meal, flour, soda, salt and baking powder. Pour into an oiled 8" x 8" baking pan. Bake in a 350 degree oven for 35- 40 minutes until lightly brown on top and toothpick inserted in center comes out clean (if you like thinner crisper bread, use larger pan). Let cool 10-15 minutes and cut in squares.

TOMATO & MOZZARELLA BAGUETTE

I had this in Paris in one of those neat street cafe's, and it tasted so fresh and good and is so quick and simple to make. Eat it with a simple meal, a steak on the grill or just alone for lunch. I hadn't had any luck finding a traditional french baguette without additives until I found one at Whole Foods Grocery Store. Totally natural, only has organic wheat flour, water, sea salt and fresh yeast, tastes GREAT.

Split baguette lengthwise in half. Cut in half again the other way. (This will make 4 open face sandwiches) Saute on low about 4 tablespoons of butter with a teaspoon of olive oil, a teaspoon of minced garlic and 2 tablespoons fresh basil. Be careful not to burn butter. Spoon on each half of bread. Slice four tomatoes and place on bread. Slice mozzarella thinly and place piece on each tomato. Broil just until cheese melts. Delicious!

Note: Adjust amount of garlic and basil to your taste. Of course, if you don't want to use the whole loaf, you can keep it for next day or freeze.

CHEESY HERB FRENCH BREAD

1 loaf	french bread (recipe on page 120 or "good" french bread)
	softened butter
	grated farmer cheese
	finely chopped fresh basil

Split bread in half lengthwise. Spread butter on both sides of bread. Lay cheese on one side along with chopped basil. Wrap tightly in foil and bake in preheated 350 degree oven for 15 minutes.

Garlic Bread:
Do the same way except instead of cheese and basil spread butter and then minced fresh garlic or garlic powder.

CRACKERS

1 cup	unbleached, all purpose flour
1 teaspoon	baking powder
1/4 teaspoon	salt
1/4 cup	butter
1/4 cup	milk

Thoroughly sift together the flour, baking powder and, salt. Cut in the cold butter until the mixture resembles coarse crumbs. Add the milk, all at once, and stir to mix. Form a ball of dough with hands. Place dough on lightly floured surface. Knead dough gently 10 strokes. Roll dough out (like pie crust). Dip a 2 or 2 ½" biscuit cutter in some flour and cut. Place dough rounds on a lightly greased (or Silpat lined) cookie sheet. Bake in a 400 degree oven for 10 minutes. Split the hot crackers with a sharp knife by holding the cracker upright with the edge on cutting board and carefully cut in half. Return cut side up crackers to same baking sheet. Bake for another 4-6 minutes until golden brown. Makes 24-30 crackers.

GRAHAM CRACKERS

These crackers are so good and easy to make. They take a little time to roll out, but well worth it. I always make a double batch and make crumbs out of some of them for pie crusts, they freeze well.

.

2 ½ cups	whole wheat flour
½ teaspoon	salt
½ teaspoon	baking powder
1/4 teaspoon	cinnamon
6 tablespoons	butter
½ cup	honey

Sift together flour, salt, baking powder and cinnamon into a bowl. Melt the butter and honey together. Pour into dry ingredients. Mix well but don't over mix or knead.. Form into several balls. Place the dough on a well floured surface and roll out a ball of dough with a well floured rolling pin. Add flour as needed if too wet. Roll out as thin as possible into a rectangle. Cut off ragged edges and cut into squares. Place 2" apart on lined cookie sheet and, using a small floured roller, roll each square again to make thinner, but don't let them tear. Prick several times with fork. Bake in a 350 degree oven for 10-12 minutes until browned. Cool on a rack.

Note: To make cracker crumbs for pie crusts, put several broken crackers in blender or food processor until you have fine crumbs. Measure crumbs and put in a plastic bag. Label the bag with how many cups, date and place in freezer. Just add melted to butter to crumbs until you have the right consistency for pie crust.

CROUTONS

2 slices	homemade bread or "good" bread
1 ½ tablespoons	butter, melted
1/16 teaspoon	garlic powder

Trim crust from bread. Cut bread into 1/2" cubes. Place in bowl. Mix butter and garlic together and pour over bread cubes. Stir gently to coat bread cubes. Spread cubes on a cookie sheet. Bake in 300 degree oven for 10-20 minutes (depending on how crunchy you want them) until dry and golden. Store, covered in the refrigerator. Sprinkle over salads or soup.

Note: You can also make these without the butter or garlic for less fat and calories.

PUMPKIN MUFFINS

1 1/4 cups	unbleached all purpose flour
2 teaspoons	baking powder
½ teaspoon	baking soda
½ teaspoon	salt
½ teaspoon	cinnamon
½ teaspoon	nutmeg
3/4 cup	mashed pumpkin (Libby's)
½ cup	brown sugar
1	egg, slightly beaten
1/4 cup	milk
1/4	canola oil
1 cup	Quaker Oats, old fashioned
½ cup	optional: dried cranberries (Sunsweet Cranberry Fruitlings) or dried cherries (Mariani)

Crumb Topping:

½ cup	brown sugar
1 tablespoon	flour
1/4 teaspoon	cinnamon
2 tablespoons	butter

Sift together flour, baking powder, soda, salt, cinnamon, nutmeg. Set aside. Combine pumpkin, brown sugar, egg, milk, oil, and oats. Blend well. Add dry ingredients all at once, and optional dried fruit, stirring just enough to moisten. Spoon batter evenly into 12 buttered muffin cups. Mix crumb topping ingredients until crumbly and sprinkle over muffins. Bake in a 400 degree oven for 18 to 20 minutes.

STREUSEL MUFFINS

1 1/3 cup	all purpose flour
1 cup	brown sugar, firmly packed
½ cup	butter, softened
2/3 cup	all purpose flour
1 ½ teaspoon	baking powder
½ teaspoon	baking soda
½ teaspoon	salt
1 ½ teaspoon	nutmeg
2/3 cup	milk
2	eggs

Combine flour and brown sugar and cut in butter until crumbly. Reserve ½ cup for topping. In the same bowl add flour, baking powder, soda, salt, nutmeg, milk and eggs. Stir just until moistened. Spoon batter evenly into 12 buttered muffin cups. Spoon on reserved topping. Bake for 18 to 22 minutes in 400 degree oven.

APPLE MUFFINS

1 ½ cups	unbleached, all purpose flour
½ cup	sugar
2 teaspoons	baking powder
½ teaspoon	salt
½ teaspoon	cinnamon
1/4 cup	butter, cold
1	egg, slightly beaten
½ cup	milk
1 cup	chopped apple (1 large)
1/4 cup	brown sugar
½ teaspoon	cinnamon

Sift together: flour, sugar, baking powder, salt and cinnamon. Cut butter into flour mixture until fine crumbs form. Mix together, egg and milk. Add milk mixture to flour mixture and stir just to moistened. Fold in apple. Spoon batter evenly into 12 buttered muffin cups. Mix together brown sugar and cinnamon and sprinkle on muffins. Bake in a 375 degree oven for 25 minutes or until golden brown.

ZUCCHINI CRANBERRY BREAD

3 tablespoons	butter, softened (not melted)
1 cup	sugar
2	large eggs
16 ounces	"good" whole berry cranberry sauce
½ cup	unsifted whole wheat flour
1 ½ cup	unsifted unbleached all purpose flour
1 teaspoon	baking soda
2 teaspoons	baking powder
2 cups	zucchini, grated

Beat butter, sugar and eggs. Stir in cranberry sauce. Fold in flour, soda and baking powder. Add zucchini. Spoon into two oiled 8" loaf pans. Bake in a 350 degree oven for 45 minutes to 1 hour or until toothpick comes out clean.

BRAN MUFFINS

1	egg, slightly beaten
1 cup	milk
2 tablespoons	butter, melted
1 cup	100% bran
1 cup	unbleached all purpose flour (or whole wheat flour)
1 tablespoon	baking powder
1/4 cup	sugar
½ teaspoon	salt

In a small bowl, mix egg, milk, butter and bran (milk should cover bran). Let stand for 15 minutes. Add flour, baking powder, sugar and salt and stir just to mix. Lightly oil 12 muffin cups. Bake in a 375 degree oven for 20 minutes

BLUEBERRY PANCAKES AND BLUEBERRY SYRUP

2 cups	unbleached all purpose flour
5 teaspoons	baking powder
½ teaspoon	salt
2 tablespoons	butter, melted
1	egg, beaten
1 cup	milk
½ cup	water (add more if you want thin pancakes)
16 ounce can	blueberries, put through a strainer and measure 1 cup liquid, if there isn't enough, add water to make 1 cup

Sift together flour, baking powder and salt. Add butter, egg, milk and water. Stir until smooth. Carefully stir in drained blueberries. Lightly oil non stick griddle. When very hot (drop of water should sizzle) spoon on batter and flip when bubbled. Spread a little butter on each pancake and serve with hot syrup.

Syrup:

2 tablespoons	flour
2 tablespoons	water
1 cup	reserved syrup
1 tablespoon	sugar

Mix flour and water together in small bowl until smooth and add to reserved blueberry syrup in pan. Add sugar, bring to a boil and simmer until thickened. Add water, if needed, to make the right consistency. Serve hot over buttered pancakes.

Note: If you have fresh blueberries, blend some of them to make liquid, and proceed with the rest of the syrup recipe.

BREAKFAST BREAD

1 ½ cups	wheat flour
1 ½ teaspoons	baking powder
½ teaspoon	cinnamon
1/8 teaspoon	nutmeg
1/4 teaspoon	salt
½ cup plus 1/8 cup	milk
½ cup	honey
1	egg, slightly beaten
1 tablespoon	oil
1 cup	apricots, dried cherries or cranberries or a combination of all or some

In a large bowl, combine flour, baking powder, cinnamon, nutmeg, and salt. In a small bowl, mix milk, honey, egg and oil. Add to flour mixture. Don't over-mix, just enough to moisten and blend. Stir in fruit. Spoon into a oiled 4" X 8" loaf pan. Bake in a 350 degree oven for 30-40 minutes or until toothpick inserted in middle comes out clean.

SAUCES AND DRESSINGS

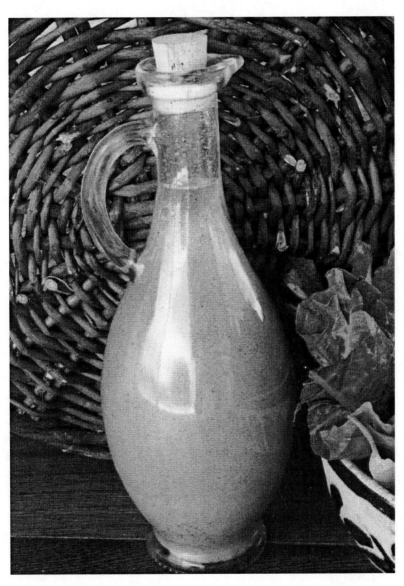

Vinaigrette #2, page 131

MAYONNAISE

This is such a easy recipe and it's great to have on hand, tastes so much better than the store bought kind

1	egg
3/4 teaspoon	salt
1 teaspoon	mustard (recipe in Sauce section of book) or dry mustard, or Robert Rothschild Raspberry Honey Mustard or Apricot Ginger
½ teaspoon	paprika
1/8 teaspoon	cayenne
2 tablespoons	apple cider vinegar
3/4 cup	olive or canola oil

In blender place egg, salt, mustard, paprika, cayenne, vinegar and 1/4 cup of the oil. Cover and switch on the motor for just a few seconds. Uncover and add the rest of the oil very gradually while the motor is running on medium or low speed. Blend until very thick and smooth (add more oil if you want thicker).

Note: Put into a glass jar with screw cap, date and refrigerate (should use within 10 days). Double or triple for potato salad, etc.

HOT MUSTARD

½ cup	dry mustard
2 tablespoons	cold water
3/4 cups	boiling water
1/4 cup	raw sugar (or try 1/8 cup honey)
2 tablespoons	apple cider vinegar (or white vinegar)
1 tablespoon	olive or canola oil
1/4 teaspoon	salt

In a bowl mix together the dry mustard and cold water to form a stiff paste. Smooth down the mixture with a rubber spatula

Pour 1/4 cup of the boiling water over the mustard, do not stir. Let the water sit on top. Allow to cool and carefully pour the water off. Pour another 1/4 cup of boiling water over the mustard and repeat the procedure. Repeat once more with the last 1/4 cup. When the last is cooled and poured off, whisk in the sugar, vinegar, oil and salt (or use mixer) and blend well. Store in a well sealed container and allow to stand overnight before using. Makes about 1 1/4 cups.

Variation to above recipe: this version is not as hot and has a nice sweet flavor:
Add 1/3 cup of pureed dried apricots (in food processor with a little water) 1/3 cup of the above mustard recipe, and 1/3 cup of honey. Cook stirring constantly over low heat for a few minutes.

SOUR CREAM SUBSTITUTE

1 cup	cottage cheese (Alta Dena Farmer Style)
1/4 cup	milk

Blend until smooth. Add seasonings to taste (salt, pepper, dill)

SALAD DRESSING

1/8 cup	basil, fresh
1/8 cup	cilantro, fresh
2 large	garlic cloves, minced
1/4 cup	olive or canola oil
1 cup	apple cider vinegar or Wild Thymes Cranberry Ginger
½ cup	rice vinegar, roasted garlic

Mix all ingredients in a jar with a tight fitting screw on lid, date and refrigerate (should use within 10 days).

HONEY VINEGAR DRESSING

1/3 cup	red raspberry or cranberry ginger vinegar (Wild Thymes)
1/3 cup	honey
1/8 teaspoon	salt
1/8 teaspoon	pepper
1 teaspoon	dry mustard
dash	nutmeg
dash	coriander

Mix all ingredients in a jar with a tight fitting screw on lid, date and refrigerate (should use within 10 days). This recipe makes enough for two large salads. Double as needed.

CREAMY SALAD DRESSING

1/4 cup	mayonnaise (recipe on page 129)
1/4 cup	creme fraiche (Vermont Butter and Cheese Company) or sour cream (Daisy)
1 teaspoon	mustard (recipe on page 129 or Rothschild) or dry mustard
1 teaspoon	vinegar, cranberry ginger balsamic (Wild Thymes)
1/4 teaspoon	horseradish (Bubbies)
1/4 teaspoon	Spice Hunter Caribbean Rub or your own mixture of seasonings

Mix all ingredients in a jar with a tight fitting screw on lid, date and refrigerate (should use within 10 days). This recipe makes enough for two large salads. Double as needed.

VINAIGRETTE

½ cup	brown rice vinegar
1/4 cup	cranberry ginger vinegar (Wild Thymes)
1/4 cup	apple juice
½ cup	olive oil
½ teaspoon	dry mustard
½ teaspoon	salt
1/8 teaspoon	pepper
1/8 teaspoon	white pepper
1/4 teaspoon	sugar

Mix all ingredients in a jar with a tight fitting screw on lid, date and refrigerate (should use within 10 days). Shake before using.

VINAIGRETTE #2

This dressing is my favorite. Its tangy and sweet and is good on any salad and you don't need to use much if you mix it very well with your salad

½ cup	apple cider vinegar
1 cup	canola or olive oil
1/4 cup	mustard (recipe on page 129 or Rothschild Raspberry Honey)
1 ½ teaspoon	salt
1 teaspoon	pepper
1/4 teaspoon	sugar

Mix all ingredients in a jar with a tight fitting screw on lid, date and refrigerate (should use within 10 days). Shake before using.

HONEY MUSTARD DRESSING

This dressing uses no oil, so there is not fat to worry about! It's very tasty and quick and easy to make

1/4 cup	honey
2 tablespoons	mustard (recipe on page 129 or Rothschild Raspberry Honey)
½ cup	rice vinegar

Mix all ingredients in a jar with a tight fitting screw on lid, date and refrigerate (should use within 10 days). Shake before using.

BARBEQUE SAUCE

2 - 28 ounce cans	tomatoes, crushed or tomato sauce (Eden Organic) or whole blended until smooth
12 ounces	tomato paste
1 teaspoon	onion salt
1 teaspoon	white pepper
1 teaspoon	cumin
1 teaspoon	dry mustard
1 teaspoon	chili powder
1 teaspoon	garlic salt or powder
3 teaspoons	salt
1/2 teaspoon	cayenne pepper
2 tablespoons	rice vinegar
1/8 cup	vinegar (Wild Thymes Cranberry Balsamic Vinegar)
½ cup	honey
1 cup	brown sugar

Combine ingredients in large saucepan and simmer for 1 hour.

Note: For variety add 1 ½ cups of fresh coconut and 1 cup of coconut milk to barbeque sauce. Simmer for about 30 minutes. Adds a nice flavor.
The easiest way to extract the milk from the coconut is to use a sharp knife and cut a hole in the top, turn it over and drain the milk out. Place the coconut on a very hard surface and smack it with a hammer to break it in half. Using a small sharp knife cut out the coconut. Use a potato peeler to get off the brown layer. In a food processor shred the coconut.

FRESH TOMATO SAUCE

I love to make this quick and easy sauce in the summer when I have fresh tomatoes and basil in my garden. It can be used in so many recipes and tastes so fresh and good.

6 cups	fresh vine ripened tomatoes, blended
2 teaspoons	salt
1 teaspoon	pepper
1/8 teaspoon	cayenne
1 tablespoon	basil, fresh, chopped
2 tablespoons	dried onion flakes

Blend tomatoes on low so you still have some chunks. Pour into saucepan and add salt, pepper, cayenne, basil and onions. Simmer on low boil for about an hour, until sauce is thickened.

Note: Use in recipes calling for homemade spaghetti sauce or pour over pasta with a little cheese grated on top for a quick, easy meal.

MARINATE FOR CHICKEN OR BEEF

This recipe makes a lot: 8 to 10 chicken breasts, thighs, large flank steak, tri tip or round steak

4 cups	water
1/4 cup	mild chili powder
½ teaspoon	cayenne
½ cup	brown sugar
1/4 cup	cilantro, fresh, finely chopped (or 1/8 cup dried)
½ tablespoon	whole coriander seed, ground
1 teaspoon	whole allspice, ground
2 tablespoons	oregano, fresh, finely chopped (or 1 tablespoon dried)
2 sprigs	mint, fresh, finely chopped
½ teaspoon	anise
1 teaspoon	coarse salt
1 tablespoon	dried onion flakes

Combine all ingredients in saucepan and simmer for 10 minutes (reserve 2 cups to serve on the side, cover and keep in refrigerator until needed). Place chicken or beef in pan only big enough for meat. Pour remaining marinade over. Cover and put in refrigerator and let sit overnight or all day. Take meat out of marinade, discard marinade. Place on foil. Grill for 10-15 minutes, each side or until done (depending on your grill)

While meat is cooking, pour the remaining 2 cups of marinade into small saucepan. Simmer for 20-30 minutes or until thickened. Serve with meat.

Serving Suggestion: Very good with baked potato, and corn.

FISH DIPPING SAUCES

1 cup	cottage cheese (Alta Dena Farmer Style)
1/4 cup	milk
1 tablespoon	dill, fresh, chopped
1/8 teaspoon	mustard (recipe on page 129, Rothschild or dry)
1/8 teaspoon	cardamom

Blend together until smooth and refrigerate until ready to serve.

Or:

4 tablespoons	creme fraiche (Vermont Butter and Cheese Co.) or sour cream (Daisy)
½ teaspoon	dill, fresh, chopped
½ teaspoon	Spice Hunter Fish Seasoning or your own combination of seasonings
½ teaspoon	mustard (recipe on page 129 or Rothschild Raspberry Honey)

Mix together until smooth and refrigerate until ready to serve

Or: Cocktail Sauce (recipe on page 151)

WHOLE BERRY CRANBERRY SAUCE

1 cup	sugar
1 cup	water
1 package	fresh or frozen cranberries

In a saucepan mix sugar and water. Stir to dissolve sugar. Bring to a boil and add cranberries. Return to a boil, reduce heat and boil gently for 10 minutes stirring occasionally. Remove from heat. Cool completely at room temperature and then refrigerate.

JELLIED CRANBERRY SAUCE

Prepare as directed above but before cooling, place a wire mesh strainer over a mixing bowl. Pour contents of saucepan into strainer. Mash cranberries with the back of a spoon scraping the outside of the strainer until no pulp is left. Stir contents of bowl, cover and cool completely at room temperature and refrigerate.

CRANBERRY APPLE RELISH

2	Granny Smith apples, finely diced
1 cup	fresh cranberries
2 stalks (1/2 cup)	celery, finely diced
1/4 cup	sugar
1/4 cup	seasoned rice vinegar
1/4 teaspoon	salt

Put all ingredients in medium frying pan. Saute over medium high heat for about 10 minutes until cranberries pop and mixture is thick. Serve hot or cold and serve with pork chops or as an accompaniment to other dishes.

GRAMP'S APPLESAUCE

My grandfather made this applesauce a couple of times a week for as long as I can remember. As soon as you walked into his house you could smell the sweet fragrance of apples and cinnamon. My kids loved it and now, I make it for my year old twin grand-daughters, Kayla and Megan who love it warm right after I make it, and my grandson Casey who is 3, loves it cold.

5 large	apples (I use Granny Smith, use your favorite)
3 tablespoons	sugar (I like to use raw sugar)
1 teaspoon	cinnamon

Place apples in pressure cooker with 1 cup water. Pressure cook for approximately 20 minutes (or according to manufacturers directions). Cool cooker, and place apples in food mill (looks like a big strainer with a blade and handle, found at any kitchen store) over large bowl. Push soft apples down with a fork and mash until all pulp is in bowl, keep turning back and forth until onlyh the skin and seeds are left in the food mill. Do one apple at a time, and after each apple clean out discards. Using 5 apples will yield about 2 cups of applesauce.Add sugar and cinnamon to apple puree in bowl and mix well. Refrigerate. Only keep a few days.

Note: This recipe is for a small pressure cooker (5 apples are the maximum that will fit). Double, etc. for the size of your cooker.

Note: If you don't have a pressure cooker, just use a large pot and add the water. You will need to check every few minutes and add water as needed. It will take about 30 minutes for the apples to get soft. A really good way of doing this is in a two piece steamer pot.

DESSERTS

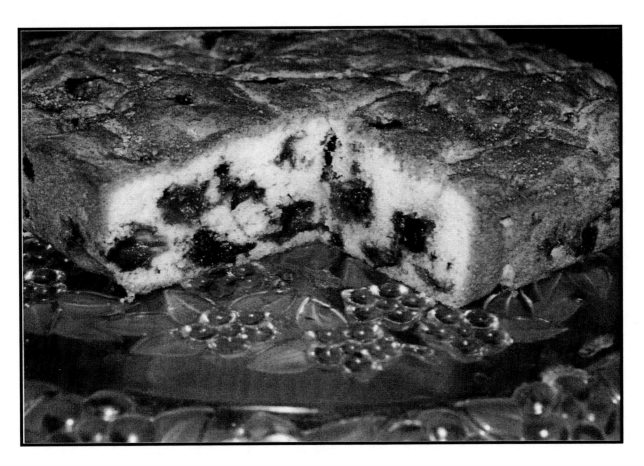

Blueberry Cake for Grampa Jerry, page 140

ANGEL CAKE, FRUIT AND WHIPPED CREAM

This is a great company dessert. For variety, check out the suggestions at the bottom of the page

1 cup	all purpose flour
3/4 cup	sugar
1 ½ cups	egg whites (12) room temperature (about ½ hour)
1 ½ teaspoons	cream of tartar
1/4 teaspoon	salt
1 ½ teaspoon	vanilla
3/4 cup	sugar

Sift flour with 3/4 cup sugar, twice. Set aside. Bowl must be completely grease free, wash until it is squeaky clean. Don't use plastic. Beat egg whites with cream of tartar, salt, and vanilla until stiff enough to form soft peaks but still moist and glossy. Add remaining 3/4 cup sugar, 2 tablespoons at a time continuing to beat until egg whites hold stiff peaks. Sprinkle 1/4 cup of flour mixture over whites, fold in. Repeat folding in remaining flour by fourths. Pour into an ungreased tube pan. Bake in a 375 degree oven for 35 to 40 minutes or until tests done. Invert pan until cool, run knife around edges and remove.

Sauce:

Drain juice from 2 cans of pitted cherries (S&W dark sweet pitted cherries) or blueberries (or fresh sliced strawberries mixed with a little sugar to make juice).Mix 2 tablespoons flour with 2 tablespoons juice in a separate bowl until smooth paste. Add gradually to the rest of cold juice in saucepan. Stir constantly over low heat until thickened. Add a little sugar or honey if you want sweeter. Add cherries or blueberries and serve over cake slices. Top with whipped cream.

WhipCream:

1 pint	heavy whipping cream (Horizon Organic)
1 teaspoon	pure vanilla
1/4 cup	sugar

Place ingredients in mixing bowl and beat until stiff peaks form.

Variations:

1. Add jelly to whipping cream instead of sugar and vanilla.

2. Cut cake in half and put half of the fruit and cream in the middle add top layer and spread with the rest of the cream and fruit.

3. My favorite way of making this cake is to use individual cake tube pans (8), put fruit in middle and cream on top. They look very elegant.

4. If you really feel ambitious, a very elegant way of serving this cake is to offer several choices of toppings. Have whipped cream in one bowl along with cherries, blueberries, strawberries, and hot carob icing (recipe in Dessert section of book) all in serving bowls so your guests can choose their favorite and make their own dessert. The individual cakes work very well with this.

ICE CREAM CAKE

4	eggs
1 1/3 cups	sugar
1 teaspoon	vanilla
½ cup	cold water
1 1/3 cups	flour
1 1/4 teaspoons	baking powder
1/4 teaspoon	salt
1 cup	powdered sugar
6 cups packed	Breyers All Natural Strawberry Ice Cream (coffee, cherry vanilla)
	Soften by placing in large bowl and stirring briskly with large wooden spoon

Beat eggs about 5 minutes at medium speed. Gradually add sugar beating constantly, add vanilla and water. Sift flour, baking powder and salt. Add sifted ingredients all at once to egg mixture blending only until batter is smooth.

Spread evenly in lightly greased parchment paper lined 10 ½" x 15 ½" x 1" jelly roll pan (deep cookie sheet). Bake about 20 minutes in a 350 degree oven or until center of cake springs back when lightly touched and light brown (don't over bake as it will not roll up right). Loosen edges and immediately turn out on towel sprinkled with about ½ cup sifted powdered sugar. Roll up, beginning at narrow end. Wrap in towel until cool (at least 1 hour). Unroll and spread softened ice cream on top and then re-roll. Sprinkle with ½ cup sifted powdered sugar. Wrap tightly in heavy duty foil and put in freezer. Slice servings, place on plates, cover with plastic wrap and let sit about 10 minutes before serving.

Serving Suggestion: For a really pretty touch, put a dollup of whipped cream mixed with Strawberry Jelly and fresh strawberries or cherries on top of each slice.

Note: Instead of ice cream, you can use whipped cream for filling (recipe in Dessert section of book under Angel Cake). Mix whipped cream with one 15 ounce can of Columbia Gorge pitted cherries, chopped (drain the juice into saucepan). Spread cream on cake and roll up, wrap and refrigerate. Drain juice of another can of cherries into saucepan, add 2 tablespoons of sugar and whisk 1/4 cup of flour into juice. Heat juice and stir until well blended and thickened. Add can of whole cherries to sauce. Serve over cake.

CARROT CAKE AND CREAM CHEESE FROSTING

This is a wonderful cake that everyone loves! It smells so good when baking!

1 cup (2 sticks)	butter
4	eggs
1 teaspoon	vanilla
2 cups	sugar
2 cups	unbleached all purpose flour
1 teaspoon	cinnamon
1 heaping teaspoon	baking soda
3 cups	grated carrots

All ingredients should be at room temperature. Butter should be soft. Put butter in mixing bowl. Add eggs one at a time, mixing well after each. Add vanilla. Sift together in large bowl: sugar, flour, cinnamon, and baking soda. Sift again. Add dry mixture a little at a time to butter mixture in mixing bowl until well blended. With large spoon fold in carrots. Oil 9" x 13" pan or two 9" cake pans and pour in batter. Bake in a 350 degree oven for approximately 40-50 minutes or until toothpick inserted in center comes at clean. Check after 30 minutes.

Frosting:

1 cup (8 ounces)	cream cheese (Gina Marie)
½ cup (1 stick)	butter
2 cups	powdered (confectioners) sugar, sifted
1 teaspoon	vanilla

Cream cheese and butter should be at room temperature. Place in mixing bowl and mix until smooth. Add vanilla. Add sugar gradually mixing until well blended. Spread frosting on cooled cake (make sure cake is cool or frosting will melt). Frosting must be refrigerated, so if you don't want to refrigerate the whole cake, frost before serving.

Note: For a sheet cake, you can cut the frosting recipe in half unless you like tons of frosting!

APPLE CAKE

2 cups	sugar
½ cup	butter
2	eggs
2 ½ cups	unbleached all purpose flour
2 ½ teaspoons	baking powder
½ teaspoon	salt
1 teaspoon	cinnamon
1 teaspoon	allspice
1 teaspoon	cloves
4 cups	chopped apples (approximately 4 large apples)

Mix sugar, butter and eggs together until creamy. Add flour, baking powder, salt, cinnamon, allspice and cloves. Stir in apples. Batter will be very stiff (I use my hands to mix in apples). Spoon into oiled tube pan (or 2 small bundt pans).Bake in a 325 degree oven for 45-60 minutes until toothpick inserted in middle of cake comes out clean. Let cool 10 minutes, run knife along edges of pan, place plate on top of cake and turn over.

Serving Suggestion: Drizzle with thin Buttercream Frosting (recipe in Dessert section of book) while warm, or sifted powdered sugar. It's also great just plain.

137

PUMPKIN CHEESECAKE

single pie crust (recipe on page 139)

16 ounces	cream cheese, softened (Gina Marie)
3/4 cup	sugar
15 ounces	pumpkin (Libbys)
1 teaspoon	cinnamon
1/4 teaspoon	ginger
1/4 teaspoon	nutmeg
2	eggs

8 ounces	heavy whipping cream, (Alta Dena) whipped with ½ teaspoon vanilla, 1/8 cup sugar until stiff peaks form

Roll and press crust onto bottom of springform pan. Put sides back on bottom. Bake in a 400 degree oven for 5 minutes. Beat cream cheese and sugar until well blended. Beat in pumpkin and spices. Add eggs one at a time, beating well after each. Pour into crust. Bake in a 350 degree oven for 50 minutes. Raise temperature to 400 degrees and bake for 10 more minutes or until toothpick comes out clean. Let cool for 10 minutes and take off sides. Store in refrigerator until serving and top with whipped cream.

PUMPKIN CAKE SQUARES

2 cups	unbleached all purpose flour
2 teaspoons	cinnamon
2 teaspoons	baking powder
1 teaspoon	baking soda
1 teaspoon	salt

4	eggs
15 ounces	pumpkin (Libby's)
1 cup	canola oil
1 2/3 cups	sugar

8 ounces	cream cheese (Gina Marie)
1/4 cup	butter, softened
2 cups	powdered sugar

Combine flour, cinnamon, baking powder, baking soda, and salt in a medium bowl. In another bowl, whisk eggs, pumpkin, oil and sugar. Stir in flour mixture. Line a 15" x 11" jelly roll pan with parchment paper or with a Silpat liner or oil pan well. Using a rubber spatula, spread the mixture evenly into pan. Bake in a 350 degree oven for 25-30 minutes until toothpick inserted in middle comes out clean. Mix cream cheese, butter and sugar until smooth. Spread on cooled cake and cut into squares.

Mix cream cheese, butter and sugar until smooth. Spread on cooled cake and cut into squares.

PIE CRUST

This recipe will make 1 large single pie crust or small 2 crust pie

1 1/4 cups	all purpose, unbleached flour
6 tablespoons	butter, cold and cut into small pieces
½ teaspoon	salt
1/4 teaspoon	sugar
1/4 cup plus 1 tablespoon	water, very cold

Place flour, butter, salt, sugar into large bowl. Cut in butter with fork or pastry blender until butter and flour form fine crumbs. Add water gradually and mix until flour just sticks together when you grab it. Don't handle it too much or it will be tough. Place dough on floured cutting board and roll out until very thin. Roll dough around rolling pin and place in pie tin. Fold under trimmed edge and use moistened fork to seal around edge of pie tin. Pierce bottom and sides of crust with fork all around (prevents puffing up). Bake in a 400 degree oven for approximately 15 minutes or until light brown.

BUTTERSCOTCH PIE

I had never had butterscotch pie until I got married and went to Kentucky. My mother-in law, Reba Bentley, who was a great country cook, made this often for her ten children. It is now my family's favorite pie (or put in custard cups for pudding)

	baked 8" pie crust, recipe above
3 tablespoons	butter
3/4 cup	brown sugar, firmly packed

In a small heavy skillet, heat butter and sugar and stir constantly over very low heat until mixture bubbles a little when you stop stirring for a second or two. Don't over cook or it will burn. Set aside.

3/4 cup	sugar
7 tablespoons	flour
1/4 teaspoon	salt
2 cups	milk
2	egg yolks (reserve whites for meringue)

Mix sugar, flour and salt together. Put milk into a medium saucepan and add flour mixture. Cook over medium heat stirring constantly until thick and bubbling. In a small bowl beat yolks slightly and add a small amount of the hot mixture and stir. Add slowly, stirring constantly to hot mixture. Add the brown sugar mixture and continue to cook and stir constantly over medium heat until it boils. Continue to cook for another minute. Put large strainer over a bowl and pour mixture through using the back of a spoon to press it through. Let cool for a few minutes and add vanilla. Cover and refrigerate for a few hours until very firm and pour into baked pie shell and top with meringue or whipped cream. For a lighter filling, mix with 1 pint of whipping cream, whipped.

Meringue:

2	egg whites
2 tablespoons	sugar

Beat egg whites with mixer and add sugar while egg whites are still frothy. Beat until stiff. Spread on filling and bake in a 350 degree oven until golden brown, about 5-7 minutes (baking meringue slowly eliminates watery meringue).

APPLE PUDDING

1/4 cup	butter, softened
1 cup	sugar
2 large	eggs, well beaten
1 ½ cups	unbleached, all purpose flour
1 teaspoon	baking soda
1 teaspoon	cinnamon
½ teaspoon	salt
2 ½ cups	apples (approximately 5) peeled, cored and grated

Beat butter and sugar with electric mixer until light and fluffy. Beat in eggs. In a medium bowl, combine flour, baking soda, cinnamon and salt. Add to butter mixture and beat until well mixed. Stir in apples. Spread mixture in a buttered 1 ½ quart mold. Cover tightly with foil. Place mold in a large pot and add water to reach halfway up sides of mold. Bring water to a boil. Cover pot. Turn down heat and simmer gently for 2 hours. Check water every 30 minutes and add boiling water as needed.

Remove pudding from pot and let cool for 10 minutes. Unmold onto serving dish. Serve warm or at room temperature.

Serving Suggestion: Tastes great with a dollup of "real" whipped cream (recipe under Angel Cake, page 135)

BLUEBERRY CAKE FOR GRAMPA JERRY

2	eggs, separated
1/4 cup	sugar
½ cup	butter
1/4 teaspoon	salt
1 teaspoon	vanilla
3/4 cup	sugar
1 ½ cups	unbleached all purpose flour
1 teaspoon	baking powder
1/3 cup	milk
2 cups	fresh blueberries, wash, remove stems and mix with 1 tablespoon of flour cinnamon sugar

Beat egg whites until stiff. Beat in 1/4 cup of sugar. In another bowl, cream butter, add salt and vanilla. Gradually add 3/4 cup sugar. Add egg yolks and beat until creamy. Sift flour with baking powder. Add alternately to creamed mixture with milk. Fold in beaten egg whites. With a large spoon, carefully fold in blueberries. Butter a 8" x 8" square pan. Spread batter in pan. Mix sugar and cinnamon together, to taste, and sprinkle on top of batter. Bake in a 350 degree oven for approximately 50 minutes or when toothpick inserted in center comes out clean.

CHEESE BLINTZES

These are wonderful for a fancy breakfast served with fresh fruit, or as an elegant dessert

Crepe Batter:

2	eggs
1 tablespoon	butter, melted
1 cup	milk
1 cup	flour
1/4 teaspoon	salt

Beat eggs, butter and milk. Add flour and salt beating until very smooth. Chill for one hour, it should be the consistency of heavy cream. If too thick, add a little milk. Grease an 8" hot <u>non stick</u> skillet with a little butter. (***or use crepe maker**) Pour 4 tablespoons of batter into the skillet turning pan to coat. Saute lightly on one side. Repeat with the remaining batter. Stack crepes on wax paper (wax paper between crepes) brown side up.

Cheese Filling:

4 ounces	cream cheese (Gina Marie)
2	egg yolks
8 ounces	Friendship Farmer cheese (soft)
2 tablespoons	sugar
1 teaspoon	vanilla

Beat filling ingredients until smooth.

Put filling on one side of crepe, fold in sides and roll up (like an egg roll). Melt butter over medium heat and saute crepes until golden brown on all sides. Serve with fresh strawberries, jam, blueberry or Cherry Sauce (recipe found in Angel Cake recipe in Dessert section of book)

Note: *I have an inexpensive crepe maker that makes paper thin crepes. If you enjoy crepes and plan to make them often, you might want to invest in a crepe maker. You can fill crepes with a variety of ingredients, be creative. They freeze very well. I double the recipe and freeze some of them. Put wax paper between them and place in a large zipper bag.

STEAMED CRANBERRY PUDDING

This is a wonderful, unusual dessert that tastes great warm or cold. With a dollup of whipped cream its extra good

1 cup	sugar
1 cup	milk
1	egg
2 tablespoons	butter, softened
2 1/4 cups	all purpose flour
1 teaspoon	baking soda
1 teaspoon	cinnamon
1 teaspoon	nutmeg
16 oz	canned whole berry cranberry sauce (365 Brand)

In mixer bowl combine sugar, milk, egg, and softened butter. Mix on medium until blended. Add flour, soda, cinnamon and nutmeg. Mix, scraping bowl often, until well blended about 2 minutes. By hand, stir in cranberries. Pour into lightly oiled 1 ½ quart mold, or casserole dish (I use a glass angel food pan). Cover tightly with aluminum foil if you don't have a tight fitting lid for your pot. Place rack (I use my stainless steel vegetable steamer) in large pot and add boiling water to just below rack. Place mold on rack. Cover and simmer (keep at a low boil) for 2 hours or until toothpick inserted in center comes out clean. Check every 20-30 minutes and add boiling water to keep water level just below rack. Remove, uncover and let stand 5 minutes.

PEACH COBBLER

3 tablespoons	butter
1 cup	flour
1/8 teaspoon	salt
1 ½ teaspoons	baking powder
1/2 cup	sugar
1/2 cup + 1 tablespoon	milk
3 cups	peeled, sliced peaches (can used "good" canned)
½ teaspoon	cinnamon
1/4 - ½ cup	sugar (to taste)
OR:	use 26 ounces of Trader Joe's Peach Sauce (don't need to add cinnamon or sugar)

Melt butter in 8"x 8" pan. Mix flour, salt, baking powder, sugar. Add milk, stir just until mixed well. Spoon batter over butter in pan.

Combine peaches, sugar, and cinnamon and pour over batter in pan.

Bake in a 350 degree oven for approximately 40 minutes or until light brown. Batter will rise over fruit as it bakes.

Note:	This makes a small cobbler, double as needed. Other fruit tastes great in this recipe also.

PUMPKIN CUSTARD

If you love pumpkin pie, you will love this custard. Warm, it tastes like pumpkin pie without the added calories of the crust. It tastes great cold also.

16 ounces	cream cheese, softened (Gina Marie)
3/4 cup	sugar
15 ounce can	pumpkin (Libbys)
1 teaspoon	cinnamon
1/4 teaspoon	ginger
1/4 teaspoon	nutmeg
2	eggs

Beat cream cheese and sugar until well blended. Add pumpkin, cinnamon, ginger, and nutmeg. Add eggs one at a time beating well after each. Pour into 8 custard cups. Place cups in baking pan and add 1" of water to bottom of pan. Bake in a 350 degree oven for 50 minutes or until firm.

Serving Suggestion: A dollup of whipped cream tastes great on this custard!

BAKED CUSTARD

I don't make this too often as it is really fattening, but so delicious!

½ cup	sugar
6	egg yolks
1½ cups	milk
½ cup	heavy whipping cream (Alta Dena)
2 teaspoons	vanilla
	nutmeg

Gradually whisk sugar into egg yolks. Gradually whisk milk, cream and vanilla into egg mixture, **except for nutmeg.** Pour into 6 custard cups. Place custard cups in a 9" x 13" pan with 1" of warm water. Sprinkle top of custard with nutmeg. Bake in a 325 degree oven for approximately 60 minutes or until knife inserted in middle comes out clean. Great warm or cold.

Note:	I save my egg yolks when I make an egg white omelet, angel cake or meringue shells, but use them within a day or two at the most.

APPLE CRISP

8 medium	apples
1/4 cup	water
1 teaspoon	cinnamon
½ cup	sugar
½ cup	flour
4 tablespoons	butter

Peel, core and dice apples and place in 9" x 13" pan with water and sprinkle with cinnamon. Blend the sugar and flour and cut in the butter until crumbly in consistency. Sprinkle over apples and bake in a 350 degree oven for 40 minutes. Broil for 5 minutes to brown on top.

SAUTEED CINNAMON APPLES

5	apples
1/4-1/3 cup	sugar
1 teaspoon	cinnamon

Peel, core and slice apples and place in medium skillet. Add sugar and cinnamon and stir. Cover and cook on medium heat for approximately 10 minutes, stirring once or twice. Uncover and cook for another 5 minutes. Makes about 2 cups.

Serving Suggestion: This is a delicious and simple dessert served over a scoop of Breyer's All Natural Vanilla Ice Cream. Also great as a side dish with pork or even for breakfast with biscuits and eggs.

POACHED PEARS

1 3/4	cups of water
½ cup	honey
2	cinnamon sticks
4	fresh pears, peeled, cored and cut in half lengthwise

Combine water and honey in a large skillet, whisk until well blended. Arrange pear halves, cut side down in a single layer in skillet. Add cinnamon sticks. Bring to a boil and simmer over low heat. Baste the pears often. Cook 30 minutes until pears are tender and the liquid is thick and reduced to about a ½ cup. Remove pears with slotted spoon and place in individual serving dishes. Discard cinnamon sticks and pour liquid over pears.

Serving Suggestion: Can serve with a scoop of Natural Breyers Vanilla ice cream placed in the center of pear.

PEAR TARTS

6	pears, peeled, cored and chopped
2 tablespoons	sugar
½ teaspoon	cinnamon

Mix the pears, sugar and cinnamon together and saute in a skillet until soft and lightly browned. Transfer to a bowl.

6 tablespoons	butter
2 teaspoons	sugar
½ teaspoons	cinnamon

| 8 slices | Oatmeal Honey Bread (recipe on page 120 or "good" bread) |

In the same skillet, over low heat, melt the butter. Add sugar and cinnamon and mix well until sugar dissolves. Cut the crust off of the bread. Cut in half, turn and cut in half again so you have 4 equal size pieces. Dip one side of each piece of bread into the butter mixture. Line the sides of giant muffin tin cups with overlapping pieces of bread with the buttered side facing out against the tin pressing as you go. Pack the pear pieces into each muffin tin until the pears are flush with the top of the tin and the bread. Bake in a 350 degree oven for about 20-25 minutes until bread is golden brown. Cool 10 minutes and carefully scoop out with large spoon onto plate. Serve immediately.

Note: You can also use fresh peaches or apples

Serving Suggestion: Great with a dollup of whipped cream or vanilla ice cream

FRUIT TARTS
This is a very easy, fast and delicious dessert

½ cup	butter
1 tablespoon	sugar
1 cup	flour

Hero Jelly: Black Cherry, Apricot or Strawberry (or other "good" jelly):

Melt butter and sugar in saucepan. Add flour immediately and stir with wooden spoon until mixture forms a ball and sides of pan are clean. Form 24 balls and place in mini muffin pan cups. Press to form crust, prick bottom with fork. Bake for 10 minutes in a 375 degree oven. Cool for 5 minutes. Turn pan over gently to release crusts. Place crusts on plate and fill with jelly. Refrigerate.

STRAWBERRY SHORTCAKE

2 pounds	(8 cups) sliced strawberries, washed and hulled
½ cup	sugar

Mix together and refrigerate.

Cake:

1/3 cup	butter, softened
3/4 cup	sugar
1 teaspoon	vanilla
2	eggs
2/3 cup	milk
1 1/4 cup	unbleached all purpose flour
2½ teaspoon	baking powder
½ teaspoon	salt

In a small mixing bowl combine butter, sugar and vanilla. Beat until combined and add eggs and then milk. Add flour, baking powder and salt. Beat on medium speed, scraping bowl often, until well mixed. Spread into oiled and floured 8" or 9" square baking pan. Bake in a 350 degree oven for 20-25 minutes or until lightly browned. Cool completely. Cut into squares. Split each square in half. Spoon strawberries and juice between squares and on top and a spoonful of whipped cream, recipe below..

Whipped Cream:

½ pint	whipping cream (Horizon)
½ teaspoon	pure vanilla
1/8 cup	sugar

Whip until stiff peaks form.

Note: You can also use biscuits instead of cake (recipe on page 122)

MERINGUE SHELLS

2	egg whites, room temperature
½ teaspoon	vanilla
1/4 teaspoon	cream of tartar
	dash of salt
½ cup	sugar

Beat egg whites, vanilla, cream of tartar and salt on high speed of mixer until soft peaks form (tips curl over). Gradually add sugar, beating until stiff peaks form (tips stand straight) and sugar is dissolved. Line a baking sheet with plain brown paper (parchment paper, or silpat liner). Using back of spoon, shape mound of meringue into shell. About 8 shells. Bake in a 300 degree oven for 35 minutes. For crisper meringues, turn off oven and leave in oven with door closed for 1 hour or a couple of hours.

Serving Suggestion: Place strawberries or any fruit mixed with a little sugar into the shell, top with Whipped Cream (recipe in Angel Cake recipe in Dessert section of book) or Breyers All Natural Ice Cream.

SUGAR COOKIES

2 1/4 cup	all purpose unbleached flour
1/4 teaspoon	salt
2 teaspoons	baking powder
½ cup (1 stick)	butter
1 cup	sugar
2	eggs, beaten
½ teaspoon	vanilla
1 tablespoon	milk

Sift together flour, salt, baking powder and set aside. Cream butter, sugar, eggs, vanilla and milk. Add flour mixture. Wrap dough in plastic wrap and put in refrigerator for an hour or overnight. Lightly flour board and rolling pin. Roll out a portion of the dough until pretty thin. Cut out cookies and place on ungreased cookie sheet. Bake in a 350 degree oven for 15-20 minutes or until edges are lightly browned.

Serving Suggestion: Frost with Buttercream Frosting (recipe below)

BUTTER CREAM FROSTING

6 tablespoons	butter, softened (not melted)
1 pound	powdered sugar (confectioners)
1/4 cup	milk
1 ½ teaspoons	pure vanilla

Mix softened butter with sugar. Add milk and vanilla gradually until very smooth.

SNOOKERDOODLES

I had never heard of these cookies, but they are my son-in-law, Brian's favorite, so I made them for him. If you like cinnamon, you'll love these cookies

2 3/4 cups	all purpose flour
2 teaspoons	cream of tartar
1 teaspoon	baking soda
1/4 teaspoon	salt
1 ½ sticks (3/4 cup)	butter, softened but not melted
1 ½ cups	sugar
2 large	eggs
1/4 cup	sugar
2 tablespoons	cinnamon

Sift together the flour, cream of tartar, baking soda, and salt. Set aside. Beat butter and sugar together until fluffy. Scrape bowl and add eggs one at a time until well mixed. Add dry ingredients and beat on low to combine. Roll dough into balls about the size of walnuts. Mix sugar and cinnamon in a bowl and roll each ball in mixture until coated. Place on greased or Silpat lined cookie sheet 2" apart and bake in a 400 degree oven for 8-10 minutes until browned but still soft.

CAROB BROWNIES

If you love chocolate like I do, but can't tolerate it (I <u>always</u> get a migraine even eating a little bit) then this is a great alternative. Very rich, full of fat, unfortunately, but oh so good (once in a while!)

1 2/3 cup	sugar
3/4 cup (1 ½ sticks)	butter, melted
2 tablespoons	water
2 large	eggs
2 teaspoons	vanilla
1 1/3 cup	flour
3/4 cup	all natural raw carob powder
1/4 teaspoon	salt
½ teaspoon	baking powder

Combine sugar, butter and water. Stir in eggs and vanilla. Sift together: flour, carob powder, salt and baking powder. Spread in 13" x 9" oiled pan. Bake in a 350 degree oven for 25 minutes or until toothpick inserted in middle comes out clean. Sprinkle with sifted powdered sugar or warm Carob Frosting (recipe on next page).

CAROB FROSTING

Spread (or heat and drizzle) this rich icing on carob brownies, yellow, white, angel cake or sugar cookies.

½ cup	sugar
3 tablespoons	carob powder
1/3 cup	milk
1/2 stick (1/4 cup)	butter
1/8 teaspoon	salt
½ teaspoon	vanilla

Mix all ingredients except vanilla in small saucepan. Bring to a boil, stirring constantly and boil for one minute. Add vanilla. Using whisk, beat until thick.

SNACKS AND APPETIZERS

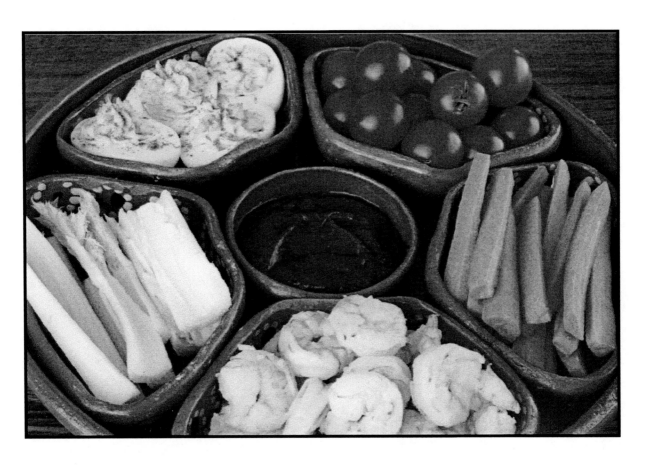

Deviled Eggs, Celery and Carrot Sticks, page 149, Shrimp Cocktail, page 151

CELERY AND CREAM CHEESE

celery   peeled, washed and dried
                            cream cheese, cottage cheese or Snofrisk cheese

Spread cheese in celery and refrigerate

CARROT STICKS

Peel and slice carrots. Great with Cream Cheese and Spinach Dip (recipe in Sauce section of book).

APPLES AND CHEESE AND CRACKERS AND CHEESE

Dip apple slices in Snofrisk cheese or spread cheese on Starr Ridge Crushed Black Pepper Crackers (or homemade crackers, recipe in Bread section of book)

DEVILED EGGS

Place eggs in saucepan with cold water at least 1 inch above eggs. Cover and bring to a boil. Take off of heat and leave, covered, in water for 15 minutes. Pour off water and replace with cold water and peel immediately. Cool in refrigerator for a few minutes. Pop out yolks into bowl and mash with fork until very fine.

Add homemade mayonnaise, mustard, (recipes in Sauce section of book) dash of tabasco, vinegar, salt and pepper to taste. Mix until pretty smooth. Using a cake decorator with a large tip squeeze into egg white shell. Sprinkle with paprika. Cover and refrigerate until ready to serve.

CUCUMBER, EGG SALAD FINGER SANDWICHES

2 large   hardboiled eggs (recipe above) peeled and finely chopped
2 tablespoons   mayonnaise (recipe in Sauce section of book)
1/8 teaspoon   salt, coarse and freshly ground pepper
4 slices   homemade bread (recipe for Honey Oatmeal Bread in Bread section of book or "good" bread, sliced thin and crust cut off)

                            cucumber slices, peeled and sliced to fit bread lengthwise

Mix chopped egg with mayonnaise and salt and pepper to taste. Spread on 2 slices of bread, top with slices of cucumber and cover with remaining slices of bread on top. Cut each sandwich into three equal fingers.

CREAM CHEESE AND SPINACH DIP

1 cup	cream cheese (Gina Marie)
1 packed cup	spinach, wash well
½ teaspoon	garlic, minced
3	sun dried tomatoes (softened in boiling water for 5 minutes)
1/4 teaspoon	salt

Put all ingredients in blender and blend on low until well mixed. Refrigerate.

Serving Suggestion: Great with "good" tortilla chips or use in Tortilla Roll-Up's (recipe on page 153). Spread on Crackers (recipe on page 125). Also good spread in celery or use for dipping carrots or other raw vegetables.

ROASTED RED PEPPER DIP

½ cup	cream cheese (Gina Marie) softened
2 tablespoons	creme fraiche (Vermont Butter and Cream Co.) or sour cream (Daisy)
3 (1/2 cup)	red peppers, de-seeded, roasted, peeled and diced
1 teaspoon	garlic, minced (extra good if you roast first, recipe on page 22)
½ teaspoon	cumin
1/4 teaspoon	salt
1/4 teaspoon	pepper

Mix all ingredients well and store in air tight container in refrigerator for 2 to 3 days.

Serving Suggestion: Great with "good" tortilla chips or use in Tortilla Roll-Ups (recipe on page 153) or spread on Crackers (recipe on page 125)

STUFFED GREEN CHILES

green chiles (Anaheim)
cream cheese (Gina Marie)

Choose green chiles that are as straight as you can get them. Cut off end and slit to the bottom. Take out white membrane and seeds. Carefully flatten and lay on foil on a cookie sheet (you want it to stay in one piece). Broil on top shelf until black, about 7-10 minutes. Place in a ziplock bag for 10-15 minutes. Take out and peel skin off. Don't wash (you wash the flavor away). Using your hands, form cream cheese the length of the chile, and place on one side of chile and roll up. Place on foil on cookie sheet, seam side down, and bake in a 350 degree oven for 20 minutes.

STUFFED TOMATO

Choose a large tomato and cut in half about and inch from the top. With a spoon, scrape out the seeds leaving a nice "bowl". Fill with tuna (recipe on page 111). Place on lettuce leaf. You can sprinkle with a little grated cheese and place under the broiler until cheese is melted.

SHRIMP COCKTAIL

1 or 2 pounds shrimp:	Peel and de-vein shrimp. In a large pot, bring water to boil. Add a tablespoon of salt. Add shrimp, bring back to boil over high heat and cook 1 minute until shrimp are pink (don't over-cook or they will be tough). Immediately drain in colander and rinse with cold water to stop the cooking process, and refrigerate.

Sauce:

1 cup	tomato sauce (Muir Glen Organic)
2 teaspoons	horseradish (Bubbies)
2 teaspoons	apricot preserves (Hero)
½ teaspoon	salt
2 tablespoons	brown sugar

Combine all ingredients in saucepan and cook until well blended and hot. Cool and refrigerate. Serve cold with cold shrimp.

Or:

1 cup	Muir Glen Organic Ketchup
4 teaspoons	horseradish (recipe in Spices and Herbs section of book)
4 teaspoons	apricot preserves (Hero)

Mix together ketchup, horseradish and preserves. Refrigerate. Serve cold with cold shrimp.

CHEESE PUFFS

1 cup	farmer's cheese, grated
1 cup	water
4 tablespoons	butter
1 teaspoon	salt
1/4 teaspoon	pepper, freshly ground
1/4 teaspoon	nutmeg, freshly ground
1 cup	unbleached all purpose flour
4 large	eggs, room temperature

In a medium saucepan bring the water, butter, salt, pepper and nutmeg to a boil. When butter has melted, take off heat and **immediately** add the flour all at once to the butter/water mixture and beat with a wooden spoon until mixture leaves the sides of the pan clean. Add the cheese and beat until well mixed. With a mixer, beat in each egg, one at a time until throughly mixed. Beat until mixture is smooth, shiny and firm.

Drop by small spoonfuls onto greased cookie sheet. Bake in upper third of the oven in a 425 degree oven for about 20 minutes or until golden and doubled in size.

Best when served right out of the oven.

Note:	These are great as an hors d'oeuvre or as an accompaniment to a first course.

FONDUE

Fondue used to be popular in the 70's and has made a real come back. It is such a great party appetizer or you can make it a meal! Fondue pots come in all sizes and price ranges. I got rather an expensive one because it has a glass liner that goes inside the pot. You put boiling water in the pot and the sterno keeps the water hot thus keeping the cheese hot all around instead of just on the bottom. I like to give each of my guests a small bowl (custard cup size or a little smaller) on a plate so they can spoon cheese into their own bowl for dipping and place their pieces of bread, veggies or fruit on the plate.

2 cups	milk
1 teaspoon	dry mustard
½ teaspoon	garlic, minced
1/4 teaspoon	pepper
½ teaspoon	salt
1/4 teaspoon	paprika
3 tablespoons	flour, unbleached all purpose
6 cups	cheese, grated (3 cups white all natural cheddar and 3 cups farmer) approximately two-8 ounce packages

In a medium saucepan over low heat, mix together milk, dry mustard, garlic, pepper, salt, paprika and flour. Stirring constantly, heat until almost boiling. Gradually stir in the cheese. Continue heating until all the cheese has melted. Don't let it boil. Pour into fondue pot and keep hot.

Note: You can also add sundried tomatoes or other herbs or spices to the sauce for variety.

Serving Suggestion: Serve with crusty bite sized pieces of french bread, broccoli, cauliflower, cucumbers, cherry tomatoes, celery, carrots, or any fresh vegetables. Also is great with apple or pear slices.

CHEESE CRISP

Lay tortilla (recipe on page 72 or "good" tortilla) on griddle or large frying pan.

Spread grated cheese on top, melt and spread with the back of a spoon.

Spread on salsa (recipe on page 73 or Pace Chunky) Roasted Red Pepper Dip, or Cream Cheese Spinach Dip (recipes on page 150).

Spoon on diced tomatoes, roasted green chili or other diced veggies. Cut with pizza cutter into wedges.

Cook until tortilla is crisp.

You can also put another tortilla on top, flip and cook on other side, to make a quesidilla.

TORTILLA ROLL-UPS

These make nice little appetizers. You can make them a few hours ahead and refrigerate. There are lots of ways to make these, some suggestions at the bottom of the recipe. This recipe is for one, double, triple, etc. for as many as you want.

1/4 cup	cream cheese (Gina Marie)
1/4 cup	creme fraiche (Vermont Butter and Cream Co.) or sour cream (Daisy)
1 tablespoon	green chiles, de-seeded, roasted, peeled, and diced
1 tablespoon	red pepper, de-seeded, roasted, peeled, and diced
1/8 teaspoon	salt
1	tortilla (recipe on page 72)

Mix softened cream cheese and creme fraiche or sour cream together and add diced green chiles, diced red pepper and salt. Spread on tortilla, do not spread too close to edges, and roll up. Wrap in plastic wrap. Refrigerate, and before serving, slice.

Variations: Another good filling is Roasted Red Pepper Dip or Cream Cheese and Spinach Dip (recipes on page 150).

Zorba's Pepperoncini's taste very good mixed with the cream cheese and creme fraiche.

You can also use a lettuce leaf, or a thin sliced piece of turkey instead of tortilla.

You can also sprinkle chopped fresh herbs on filling, such as: basil, dill, oregano, etc.

PIZZA CRUST

3/4 cup	water
2 tablespoons	canola oil
2 cups	all purpose flour or bread flour
½ teaspoon	sugar
2 teaspoons	salt
2 teaspoons	active dry yeast

Bread machine: (dough setting). Add water, oil, flour, sugar and salt to pan. Tap to settle dry ingredients. Make a slight well in center of dry ingredients and add the yeast. When timer goes off, remove bread placing on floured surface.* Knead about 1 minute and then let it rest for 15 minutes. Roll dough out to fit 12 or 14" oiled pizza pan (I put the ball of dough right in the middle of the pan and use a small roller and roll to fit. I also like to use stoneware, makes a very crispy crust). Press dough into pan forming an edge. Let dough rise in a warm, draft free place for 20-25 minutes. Spread sauce (recipes on following pages) evenly over crust and top with cheese. Bake in preheated 425 degree oven for 20-25 minutes or until crust is done (bottom rack of the oven). Let rest 5 minutes before cutting.

Oven method:

Mix water, oil, flour, sugar and salt. Add the yeast. Knead for 5 minutes. Let rise for 60 minutes in draft free place. * use directions above.

Note: If you like a really thin crust, divide dough in half and roll on pizza pan with small roller. Make two pizzas or put the other half of dough in large zipper bag and use in the next day or two.

PIZZA

1	pizza crust (recipe on page 153)
1 ½ cups	sauce (recipe below), or Eden Organic Pizza/Pasta Sauce or Sassafras Red Pepper Pizza Sauce (can add 1 pound of browned lean ground beef or "good" sausage to sauce)
1 cup	grated mozzarella cheese or farmer cheese

Saute beef until brown and drain off liquid. Add sauce and simmer for a few minutes. Spoon mixture on un-baked pizza crust and bake in a 425 degree oven for 20-25 minutes or until crust is done. Let rest for 5 minutes before cutting.

Sauce:

1 pound	ground sirloin or very lean ground beef
1/4 cup	dried onion flakes
2 tablespoons	oregano, fresh (or 1 tablespoon dried)
1 teaspoon	salt, coarse
1 teaspoon	garlic, minced
6 ounces	tomato paste
1 cup	water

Saute beef until brown and drain off liquid. Add onion, oregano, salt, and garlic. Stir in tomato paste and then add water. Simmer for a few minutes on low, stirring often.

Note: You can also use homemade spaghetti sauce (recipe in Pasta section of book). Spread on the crust and sprinkle with cheese and bake.

GARDEN PIZZA

I love to make this delicious pizza in the summer when I have all my fresh vegetables and herbs

1	pizza crust (recipe in Snack section of book)
3 tablespoons	butter
1 tablespoon	garlic, minced
3 tablespoons	basil, fresh, chopped (or 1 tablespoon dried)
1-2 cups	tomatoes, fresh, cut in half, scoop out seeds (discard) and chop the meaty part (you don't want the tomatoes to be liquidy as it makes the crust soggy)
1-2 cups	peppers (red, green, yellow) de-seeded, roasted, peeled, and diced
1-2 cups	farmers or fresh mozzarella cheese, grated

Melt butter in small frying pan. Add garlic and stir a few times, add basil.

Bake pizza crust for 10 minutes. Take out and immediately, spread on the garlic and basil. Spoon on the tomatoes and peppers. Sprinkle on the cheese. Bake for 10-15 minutes in a 425 degree oven until bubbly.

Note: Use any other fresh herbs or garden vegetables that you may have. You can also use roasted garlic (recipe in Kitchen Techniques section of book) and spread on crust. Saute herbs in a little butter and spread over the garlic, then tomatoes and cheese.

HEALTHY SNACK BARS

I wanted to come up with a no fat protein bar without too much sugar that I could eat on the run for an energy boost or for a quick breakfast. Of course, these don't taste like a high fat, high sugar muffin, but I like them a lot

1/4 cup	light brown sugar, packed
1/4 cup	honey
1/3 cup	applesauce (recipe on page 134 or "good" applesauce)
½ cup	milk (or use 2/3 cup of applesauce and eliminate the milk)
1 teaspoon	pure vanilla extract
2 large	egg whites
3/4 cup	whole wheat flour
2 teaspoons	baking powder
1/4 teaspoon	baking soda
1/4 teaspoon	salt
1/4 teaspoon	nutmeg
1 ½ teaspoons	cinnamon
1 ½ cups	old fashioned oats or granola (or ½ of each)
1/4 cup	wheat germ
1/4 cup	oat bran
2 tablespoons	vegetarian rice protein
1 cup	shredded carrot
½ cup	dried cherries or cranberries (unsulfured)
½ cup	dried apricots (unsulfured) finely chopped
1 cup	apple, finely diced

Mix sugar, honey and applesauce until well blended. Add milk, vanilla and egg whites.
In another bowl, sift together flour, baking power, soda, salt, nutmeg, and cinnamon. Add oats, wheat germ, oat bran and rice protein. Add to sugar mixture along with carrots, cherries, apricots and apple. Stir just until well blended.

Lightly oil 9" x 13" baking pan and spoon batter into pan. Bake in a 350 degree oven for 25- 30 minutes or until a wooden pick comes out clean

Note: If you don't like one of the fruits or carrots, just double up on the one that you do like or any combination of fruit amounting to 3 cups.

PROTEIN DRINK

I drink this in the morning or have it for a mid-day snack for an energy boost

2 tablespoons	vegetarian rice protein
1 cup	strawberries, frozen, cut up (or other frozen fruit)
1 cup	milk
1 tablespoon	wheat germ
1 tablespoon	strawberry or apricot preserves (Hero brand) or honey

Place all ingredients in blender and blend until smooth
Or: 2 cups frozen fruit, 2 tablespoons protein powder, 1 tablespoons wheat germ, 1 cup of juice (apricot, apple, peach, etc.) or water (add a little honey to make sweeter).

GRANOLA

3 cups	old fashioned rolled oats
½ cup	wheat germ
1/4 cup	oat bran
1/4 cup	whole wheat flour
3 tablespoons	brown sugar, packed
2 teaspoons	cinnamon
1/4 teaspoon	nutmeg
1/4 teaspoon	ginger
½ teaspoon	salt
1-2 cups	dried cranberries (or any other combination of dried fruit that you like)
½ cup	pure 100% apple juice
3 tablespoons	honey, warmed
1 tablespoon	pure vanilla
2 tablespoons	butter, melted

Combine the oats, wheat germ, oat bran, flour, brown sugar, cinnamon, nutmeg, ginger, salt and cranberries. In a small bowl whisk the juice, honey, vanilla and butter. Add to the dry ingredients. Mix well. Spread the mixture onto a buttered, oiled, or Silpat lined baking sheet. Bake in a 300 degree oven for approximately 40-45 minutes, stirring well every 15 minutes. It will be brown and dry to the touch, but be careful not to over cook. Cool on baking sheet. Store in an airtight container.

BREAD MACHINE SOFT PRETZELS

1 cup plus 2 tablespoons	water (warm, but not hot)
3 cups	all purpose flour
3 tablespoons	brown sugar
1 ½ teaspoons	active dry yeast
2 quarts	water
½ cup	baking soda
	coarse salt

Place the water, flour, sugar and yeast in bread machine. Select the dough setting. Check the dough after 5 minutes of mixing and add water or flour if necessary. When dough is finished, place dough onto a lightly floured surface. Divide dough into 8 balls. With your fingertips, roll each ball into a 20" rope. Form a circle and pull each end down and cross over to make a pretzel shape. Squeeze dough together to attach. In a large pot bring water and baking soda to boil. Carefully drop pretzels into boiling water, 2 at a time. Boil 15 seconds. Remove with a slotted spoon to a paper towel lined plate. Place boiled pretzels on buttered baking sheets. Bake in a 425 degree oven for 8-10 minutes or until golden brown. Lightly brush with water and sprinkle with salt. You can also sprinkle them with cinnamon sugar.

INDEX OF RECIPES

INDEX OF RECIPES

PORK

FISH

MEXICAN

PASTA DISHES

EGG DISHES

SIDE DISHES

VEGETABLES

SALADS

SOUP

BREADS, ROLLS, BISCUITS, MUFFINS, PANCAKES, CRACKERS, CROUTONS

SAUCES and DRESSINGS

DESSERTS

SNACKS & APPETIZERS

ISBN 155395290-1

9 781553 952909